ETHICAL DILEMMAS
IN NEUROLOGY

Volume 36 in the Series

Ethical Dilemmas in Neurology
ADAM ZEMAN, MA, MRCP, DM
LINDA L EMANUEL, MA, MD, PhD, FACP
Consulting Editors

OTHER MONOGRAPHS IN THE SERIES

ETHICAL DILEMMAS IN NEUROLOGY

ADAM ZEMAN
Consultant Neurologist
Department of Clinical Neurosciences
University of Edinburgh, Western General Hospitals, Edinburgh

LINDA L EMANUEL
Vice President Ethics Standards
American Medical Association, Chicago, Illinois

W.B. Saunders Company
London · Edinburgh · New York · Philadelphia · St Louis · Sydney · Toronto · 2000

WB SAUNDERS
An imprint of Harcourt Publishers Limited

© Harcourt Brace Publishers 2000

⊠ is a registered trademark of Harcourt Brace and Company Limited

The right of Adam Zeman and Linda L Emanuel to be identified as authors of this work has been asserted by them in accordance with the Copyright, Designs and Patents Act 1988

First published 2000

ISBN 0-7020-22276

British Library Cataloguing in Publication Data
A catalogue record for this book is available from the British Library

Library of Congress Cataloguing in Publication Data
A catalog record for this book is available from the Library of Congress

Note
Medical knowledge is constantly changing. As new information becomes available, changes in treatment, procedures, equipment and the use of drugs become necessary. The editors/authors/contributors and the publishers have, as far as it is possible, taken care to ensure that the information given in this text is accurate and up-to-date. However, readers are strongly advised to confirm that the information, especially with regard to drug usuage, complies with the latest legislation and standards of practice.

Commissioning Editor: Miranda Bromage
Project Managers: Claire Brewer, Susan Rana
Production Manager: Mark Sanderson

The
publisher's
policy is to use
paper manufactured
from sustainable forests

Typeset by IMH (Cartrif), Loanhead, Scotland
Printed and bound in China

Contents

Series Editor's Foreword

Ethics is the single aspect of medicine most likely to cause sleepless nights in physicians' and surgeons' homes. Situations in which one moral principle conflicts with another occur much more often than anticipated by medical students, or by outsiders. Neurologists and neurosurgeons bear an even greater share of these challenges than many other disciplines. The most obvious reason is that diseases of the nervous system may affect mental functions, especially consciousness and communication. Yet other neurological disorders such as paralysis, involuntary movements or epilepsy may impair a patient's lifestyle or even dignity to almost the same degree.

True enough, it is the physicians' duty to serve their patients' interests first and foremost. The demands of third parties are dutifully swept aside. But real problems arise when the patient's interest is at odds with a second ethical imperative: the obligation to speak the truth, to respect the patient's autonomy, to preserve life, to obey the law, or to serve interest of society at large. Sometimes it is not even clear who 'the patient' is: the intact individual who made out advance directives in the past, or the intellectually damaged person who is in this bed now. Answers to all these questions are not uniform. They change with time (telling patients they had cancer was regarded a heroic act 30 years ago), and with culture (even within Western Europe the potentially rival claims, in the face of terminal disease, of patient autonomy and the sanctity of life are giving rise to a range of solutions).

This book is designed to guide the neurologist and the neurosurgeon through the most common minefields of morality, by offering solutions or at least by clarifying the options. Because each of these situations requires specific expertise, it consists of a series of essays by different authors - a departure from the usual format in this book series. Yet the editors, Dr Adam Zeman (British neurologist) and Linda Emanuel (American ethicist) have done their best to ensure coherence and complementarity. The neurological community is indebted to them and the authors for having provided this unique book.

JAN VAN GIJN

Foreword

Medicine has changed radically in the past two decades. As Sir Cyril Chantler has put it: 'Medicine used to be simple, ineffective and relatively safer. It is now complex, effective, and potentially dangerous. The mystical authority of the doctor used to be essential for practice. Now we need to be open and work in partnership with our colleagues in health care and our patients'. (Quoted in *A New Medical Ethic Needed*. Editorial in the *Guardian*, 23 November 1998).

Of no branch of medicine is this more true than neurology. Greatly widened therapeutic options offer the possibility sometimes of cure, often of prolonging life. But many new treatments carry risks and the effectiveness of some is at best modest so that improvement in the quality of life is problematic, many are expensive. How should decisions be made about what treatments are to be available, who should receive them, and at what stage of the illness? Genetic diagnosis of untreatable conditions such as Huntington's disease – with profound implications both social and medical for the individual and the family – can now be made before symptoms develop. When should it be? Who should be told? The final stages of some illnesses – e.g. motor neurone disease – are dreadful. How should the end be anticipated, and how managed?

These are but some of the new range of ethical dilemmas which confront the contemporary neurologist. This book will be an invaluable guide. The contributors cover not only many of the practical issues that we face day by day, but also the philosophical approach to ethics which will help the practitioner to see more clearly the problems presented by individual patients and provide a basis for a balanced solution of them.

Dr Zeman and his colleagues are to be congratulated on their timely contribution to a topic of profound importance.

IAN McDONALD

Preface

The editors of this volume were colleagues at a British medical school 20 years ago. We shared an interest in neurology. One of us (LE) crossed the Atlantic, trained as a physician, and then pursued a growing preoccupation with ethics into a full-time career as a medical ethicist. The other (AZ) became a clinical neurologist. We have been delighted to have an opportunity to collaborate in a project which marries medical ethics to clinical neurology, exploring some of the ethical dilemmas which neurologists encounter in their everyday practice.

Transatlantic collaboration has proved trickier at times than we might have expected. Britain and America are indeed divided by a common language. But we believe that this book has been enriched by the geographical and intellectual range of its contributors, who include clinicians, specialists in medical ethics and professional philosophers. We are very grateful to them all for their hard work on their chapters.

We are grateful also to Charles Warlow for mooting the idea in the first place, to Sean Duggan at WB Saunders for keeping us up to the mark and to Gill Robinson and Miranda Bromage for their editorial guidance. Ann Dearie, Rosemary Anderson, Deidre Davidson, Katherine Rouse and Shannon Smith have provided cheerful and efficient secretarial help, refusing to accept defeat at the hands of the unruliest fax machine. Our families have put up with an extra distraction from duties at home and our final thanks are to them.

ADAM ZEMAN
LINDA L EMANUEL

Authors

David Bates MA, MD, BChir, FRCP
Consultant Neurologist and Senior Lecturer in Neurology, University of Newcastle upon Tyne, UK

Jessica Wilen Berg JD
American Medical Association, Institute for Ethics, Chicago, Illinois, USA

Rebecca Dresser JD
Professor, School of Law and Program for the Medical Humanities, School of Medicine, Washington University, St Louis, USA

Linda L Emanuel MA, MD, PhD, FACP
Vice President Ethics Standards, American Medical Association, Chicago, Illinois 60610, USA

Grant Gillett FRACS, DPhil (Oxon)
Professor of Biomedical Ethics, University of Otago; Department of Neurosurgery, University of Otago and Dunedin Hospital, Dunedin, New Zealand

Anthony C Grayling, MA, DPhil (Oxon)
Lecturer in Philosophy, Birbeck College, University of London: Supernumerary Fellow of St Anne's College, Oxford, UK

Tony Hope MA, PhD, MB BCh, FRCPsych
Reader in Medicine and Honorary Consultant Psychiatrist, Division of Public Health and Primary Care, University of Oxford, UK

Thomas G Horejsi BA
Medical Student, University of Minnesota Medical School, Minneapolis, USA

Robert Howard MA, MD, MRCPsych
Senior Lecturer and Consultant in the Psychiatry of Old Age, Institute of Psychiatry, London, UK

Edmund G Howe MD, JD
Professor of Psychiatry, Director, Program in Ethics and Associate Professor of Clinical Medicine, Uniformed Services University of the Health Sciences, Bethesda, USA

Richard I Lindley MD, FRCP (Edin)
Senior Lecturer, Department of Clinical Neurosciences, The University of Edinburgh, Western General Hospitals, Edinburgh, UK

Calixto Machado MD, PhD
Institute of Neurology and Neurosurgery, Ciudad de la Habana, Cuba

Diane E Meier MD
Professor, Departments of Geriatrics and Medicine; Director, Palliative Care Program and Catherine Gaisman Professor of Medical Ethics, Mount Sinai School of Medicine, New York, USA

Philip R Muskin MD
Chief, Consultation-Liaison Psychiatry, Columbia Presbyterian Medical Center, New York; Associate Professor of Clinical Psychiatry, Columbia University, College of Physicians and Surgeons; Faculty Psychoanalyst, Colombia University Psychoanalytic Center for Training and Research, New York, USA

Hattie Beth Myers PhD
Member, Institute for Psychoanalytic Training and Research (IPTAR) and International Psychoanalytic Association (IPA), on faculty in IPTAR's training program, New York, USA

Peter Singer MA (Melb), BPhil (Oxon)
DeCamp Professor of Bioethics, Princeton University, Princeton, New Jersey, USA

Christopher David Ward MD, FRCP
Head, Division of Rehabilitation and Ageing, University of Nottingham; Honorary Consultant in Rehabilitation Medicine and Neurology, Derbyshire Acute Hospitals, UK

Charles P Warlow MD, FRCP
Professor of Medical Neurology, Department of Clinical Neurosciences, The University of Edinburgh, Western General Hospitals, Edinburgh, UK

Simon Wessely MA, MSc, MD, FRCP, FRCPsych
Professor of Epidemiological and Liaison Psychiatry, Department of Psychological Medicine, King's College School of Medicine and Institute of Psychiatry, London, UK

Ian R Williams MB ChB, FRCP
Consultant Neurologist, The Walton Centre for Neurology and Neurosurgery, Liverpool, UK

Susan M Wolf JD
Associate Professor of Law and Medicine, Center for Biomedical Ethics, University of Minnesota Law School, Minneapolis, USA

Adam Zeman MA, MRCP, DM
Consultant Neurologist, Department of Clinical Neurosciences, University of Edinburgh, Western General Hospitals, Edinburgh, UK

Introduction

ETHICAL DILEMMAS

He who saves a single life, saves the world entire.
Talmud, Sanhedrin 37a

Don't just do something—stand there!
Advice from a wise physician

Two medical stereotypes coexist in the public mind, among other, less flattering versions. One portrays the doctor as a steely-nerved technician, steering patients expertly through the dangerous waters of their illnesses, tweaking an instrument here, adjusting an infusion rate or a ventilator setting there. The aim of the exercise—saving life—is simple and unambiguous; the means are complex and dauntingly scientific. Television delights in real and fictitious examples of this incisive figure. The second stereotype depicts a seasoned physician who long ago learned the hard lesson that most of our ills have no technical solutions. This somewhat dog-eared and disillusioned medic can more often offer wisdom than a cure, but her counsel is nonetheless a comfort to her patients.

There is, of course, some truth in both of these stereotypes. Modern medicine demands technical expertise and a solid base of evidence. But any clinical neurologist who reflects on last week's work is likely to agree that the really tricky problems were as often ethical as scientific—concerning what ought to be done, rather than how to do it. Here are a few examples of these everyday ethical dilemmas.

I am assessing a patient with early dementia in the clinic. She has told me that she dreads the diagnosis of Alzheimer's disease. Should I tell her that, in all likelihood, this is precisely the problem?

A father of three young children fulfils the indications for the use of beta-interferon in multiple sclerosis. He is likely to lose his job when he next relapses and insists that he wishes to take this drug. I am persuaded that the drug has some efficacy but accept that it is hugely expensive for the health gain purchased. Should I fight my patient's cause with the Health

Board, who do not wish to fund it, or bow to the argument of the health economists, and avoid writing this controversial prescription?

We admit a patient with massive bilateral cerebral infarcts and severe pneumonia. The prognosis is dire. I very much doubt that attempts at curative treatment are in her best, interests, or those of her family, but her husband wishes us to 'pull out all the stops' and intervene aggressively. Should we?

A young mother of two children continues to drive ('only short distances and only very occasionally') despite her undoubted temporal lobe epilepsy, with minor seizures once a month. She repeatedly fails to inform the licensing authority, despite my urging. Should I breach confidence and do so myself?

A woman in her forties is losing the use of her legs and losing control of her bladder because of spondylotic cord compression. She is terrified of hospitals and declines treatment. I explain the likely outcome. Is there anything else I can or should do?

I am a full time employee of the National Health Service. I am invited to spend a few hours each week seeing patients in the local private hospital in the evening— for a fee. They will be seen sooner and more thoroughly than my other patients, on the basis of wealth rather than need. Is it ethical to accept this invitation?

A man in the later stages of motor neurone disease, miserable and uncomfortable, asks me to speed his end. His family is distraught about his suffering. Should I accede to his request?

A patient is admitted acutely after a stroke. I am tempted to follow the standard line of conservative management. But a trial of thrombolytic therapy has recently been mounted in my hospital. Entering patients requires form-filling, discussion of consent, randomization calls, etc., and I have other things to do. Is there any ethical imperative to find the time to enter this patient in the trial?

Dilemmas like these are the everyday business of medicine. But as neither the dictates of law nor the urgings of morality give unequivocal guidance, such questions are peculiarly difficult to resolve. They excite strong emotions, and it is often impossible to arrive at solutions which satisfy all concerned. Until recently, medical education avoided this uncertain territory, and many of us feel ill-equipped to deal with it. Yet we ignore it at our peril. Issues of communication, consent and confidentiality, of the rationing of health care and treatment towards the end of life, matter enormously to our patients and their families. Dissatisfaction with doctors often stems as much from our failure to deal thoughtfully with these problems as from our technical shortcomings.

This book was conceived with the aim of assisting in the critical thinking that neurologists and their colleagues must engage in as they face the ethical dilemmas which occur in everyday practice. It is not a systematic textbook of neurological ethics. Instead we have invited clinicians (twelve of our eighteen authors) and academics of various backgrounds, from England, the United States and elsewhere, all with an interest in medical ethics, to reflect on some of the common dilemmas in the clinic and the ward. We have encouraged our authors to illustrate their essays with clinical examples. Where legal rulings and empirical research bear on the ethical issues, we have encouraged our contributors to discuss them even though they may not be applicable throughout the world.

Common sense is arguably the most important aid of all in negotiating the minefield of ethical debate. We hope that these essays will enable our readers to test and fortify professional common sense. If they help us, as physicians, to scrutinize aspects of our practice which we normally gloss over, and to question some familiar 'certainties', then they will have done their work.

THE CONTRIBUTIONS

The subject of ethics is so unfamiliar to many doctors that we decided to begin the book with an accessible contribution from a professional philosopher. Anthony Grayling is a philosopher of logic and language. His essay sketches the history of ethics in the Western philosophical tradition and introduces the concepts which subsequent contributors apply to specific dilemmas. He acknowledges the difficulties in applying ethical theories to practical problems, but argues that gaining some acquaintance with the range of ethical opinion will enhance the quality of our day-to-day clinical decisions.

The cluster of essays that follow discuss matters of diagnosis and communication.

The opening contributions by Rebecca Dresser and by Susan Wolf and Thomas Horejsi examine the easily neglected issue of pre-test counselling: when should clinicians seek consent to make a diagnosis?

It is understandable that hard-pressed physicians are sometimes impatient with the demand that they should counsel their patients before investigating them. But Rebecca Dresser endorses the arguments for the view, now broadly accepted, that consent should, where possible, be sought before performing an HIV test. Neurologists who are persuaded by these arguments might ask themselves whether they apply only to the diagnosis of HIV. If the 'potential burden' of a positive HIV test is sufficiently heavy to warrant pre-test counselling, should doctors not be offering something similar to patients before we embark, for instance, on the investigation of multiple sclerosis?

More genes are expressed in the central nervous system than in any other organ, and neurogenetics is one of the major growth points in clinical neurology. Susan Wolf reviews the genetic diagnosis of Huntington's, Tay–Sach's and Alzheimer's disease, closing with a series of recommendations for the use and regulation of genetic tests for neurological disorders. The need for counselling asymptomatic individuals at risk is generally accepted: Susan Wolf advises that doctors should offer a similar service to suspected symptomatic sufferers.

Wolf and Dresser tackle ethical issues which arise before we request a diagnostic test. In the second pair of essays, two psychiatrists, Simon Wessely and Robert Howard, whose special interests lie in areas of overlap between neurology and psychiatry, discuss the tricky question of whether diagnoses should always be disclosed.

Simon Wessely considers how to set about explaining a diagnosis of hysteria or chronic fatigue syndrome. Most neurologists will have discovered that, while they are sometimes tempting, confrontation and accusation tend to be unproductive strategies in the management of these disorders. But how can doctors combine honesty about the diagnosis they suspect with sufficient tact to retain their somatizing patients' trust and cooperation? Simon Wessely reminds us gently of our duty to 'do no harm', invites us to question our own assumptions about the nature of these illnesses, and recommends a pragmatic approach to deciding what to tell.

Robert Howard discusses the issue of breaking the diagnosis of dementia. Most people report that they would want to be told the news if they developed dementia themselves, while at the same time preferring that their relatives are not told when they actually fall prey. Robert Howard argues that the diagnosis should, where possible, be shared—accepting that severe cognitive impairment and psychological vulnerability will sometimes countervail this advice.

However they have made a diagnosis and conveyed it to the patient, doctors generally accept their obligation to ensure that it remains confidential. But the duty to maintain confidentiality is not absolute. When should it be breached? Concealment of diagnoses sometimes has pernicious effects on public health and public safety. Jessica Berg outlines the ethical and legal considerations which apply to this dilemma. Indicating when the interests of an individual third party, or of a population, might overpower the primary commitment to patient confidentiality, Jessica Berg suggests some guidelines for prudent reporting.

Diagnosis has traditionally been the neurologist's forte, but neurologists now have powerful treatments at their disposal as well. The second cluster of essays discusses ethical dilemmas raised by researching, rationing and enforcing treatment.

The movement for 'evidence-based medicine' is enjoying its heyday. Charles Warlow and Richard Lindley are enthusiastic proponents of the need to base our day-to-day practice on conclusive evidence rather than on tradition or 'expert opinion'. Doctors can only hope to achieve this if they gather the evidence themselves, and Warlow and Lindley hope to persuade you of your duty to participate in high-quality clinical trials. They discuss the ethical dilemmas which arise in the conduct of such trials, arguing that where the science is sound the ethics should more or less look after themselves.

It was not easy to show that aspirin is effective in the prevention of transient ischaemic attacks (Antiplatelet Trialists' Collaboration, 1994) Establishing which types of surgery for cervical myelopathy are effective for which groups of patients poses even more daunting problems. Grant Gillett, a neurosurgeon with a background in philosophy, discusses the special difficulties in testing neurosurgical techniques. He argues that considered clinical judgement retains an important role in the development of therapy even if, as Hippocrates wrote, it 'sometimes fails in exactness'.

Advances in basic neuroscience have spawned a new generation of drugs and underlined the vexed dilemma of how to ration scarce resources. These drugs—which include riluzole for motor neurone disease (Bensimon *et al.*, 1994), the beta-interferons for multiple sclerosis (IFNB Multiple Sclerosis Study Group, 1993) and the growing family of acetylcholinesterase inhibitors for

Alzheimer's disease (Coney-Bloom *et al.*, 1998; Rogers *et al.*, 1998)—have several features in common. All appear to have proven efficacy in clinical trials. In each case, it is controversial whether this measurable effect translates into a really useful health gain. Every one of these drugs is expensive, and together these agents threaten to consume large parts of existing drug budgets. Who then should receive these treatments? Who should decide? David Bates, a British neurologist who has extensive experience in the treatment of multiple sclerosis, tackles the issue of beta-interferon.

Tony Hope addresses another familiar treatment dilemma. There is sometimes no doubt in our minds about the appropriate management of a patient's disorder, and no difficulty in mobilizing the resources the treatment requires, but the patient can not or will not give consent. Consent may be lacking because a patient is incompetent to give it—perhaps delirious, demented or psychotic—or because he or she is simply unwilling to accept our rational advice. With the help of several case examples, Tony Hope analyses the legal and ethical grounds for enforcing treatment. These will not always empower us to administer the treatment we might wish to give: on occasion we must respect decisions we regard as foolish or misguided.

Peter Singer brings a professional philosopher's logic to the questions of embryo and animal rights. One major ethical tradition, to which Peter Singer's work belongs, locates the basis for ethical judgement in the tendency of actions to promote pleasure or to prevent pain. On this kind of view, sentience is the source of moral value. Singer's essay applies this tradition to the ethics of animal and embryo research, concluding that work with animals is *less* easily defensible than research using human embryos. Readers who disagree may nonetheless find their intuitions severely tested by Singer's arguments.

Doctors are not always detached observers of the moral scene. Medicine is our livelihood and conflicts of interest can easily arise. The following two chapters discuss two dilemmas of this kind.

Ian Williams brings his experience of helping in the expansion of neurological services in the North West of England to bear in his topical essay. Written during the fiftieth anniversary of the NHS, he asks whether private practice complements or threatens public service. He concludes that, in the British system, where the great majority of private practitioners also work in the state sector, the net effect of private practice is detrimental to public health. This debate raises fundamental questions about human motivation. Public service presupposes the willing participation of public servants. It must be in the interests of public health that the professional and financial rewards for practising medicine should be sufficient to recruit the doctors of the future. The next millennium is sure to see continuing controversy about which mix of public and private provision maximizes proper motivation and health gain.

Edmund Howe considers the conflicts of interests which can arise when a doctor owes a duty of allegiance to his military superiors as well as a duty of care to his patients. The controversial subject of 'Gulf War Syndrome' provides his test case. The Gulf War confronted military medics with a succession of scientific and ethical dilemmas: who should receive a limited supply of a vaccine with side-effects which were poorly known but which might prove life-saving on the battlefield? What should soldiers be told about the potential threats from chemical pollution during the War? And in its aftermath, how should sufferers from the Gulf War Syndrome be counselled about their mysterious disorder?

The closing essays concern the end of life. This, needless to say, comes to us all, but many doctors are uncomfortable in the ethical hinterland of death. These four essays pick out questions with which neurologists often have to grapple.

Techniques of intensive care have made it possible to survive illnesses which were once invariably fatal. Many of our patients are extremely grateful to them. But these same techniques have created possibilities for prolonging badly damaged lives which some people find disturbing. Advance directives, or living wills, were devised to enable individuals to influence their future management in circumstances in which they cannot state their wishes. Some people are reassured by this extension of their current autonomy into an uncertain future, but, as the examples in Linda Emanuel's essay make clear, interpreting a living will may not be plain sailing. It requires a thoughtful assessment of a patient's present state as well as of her past wishes. Nonetheless, the process of planning has proven surprisingly helpful to patients, families and clinicians alike.

Sometimes doctors have to ask themselves whether active treatment is achieving anything worthwhile. Chris Ward, a specialist in neurological rehabilitation, considers the principles which should guide doctors when we weigh up the pros and cons of continued curative treatment. His examples remind us that our professional perceptions of the quality of a life can differ sharply from the perceptions of the patients and family. Our 'intuition' is a necessary but insufficient guide.

Many doctors may be willing to withdraw treatment which has become futile. But as a general rule doctors hesitate to take deliberate measures to expedite death. If we refuse to do so, we sometimes come into direct conflict with the autonomy of a patient who wishes us to end his or her life. Diane Meier draws on her own and others' experience of terminal care in considering the motives which might be at work in a doctor who has been asked to hasten death. With her co-authors, Hattie Myres and Phillip Muskin, Diane Meier makes a compassionate case that doctors should continue to strive to be advocates for life.

Calls from Intensive Care to assist in the diagnosis of brain death are among the grimmer aspects of a neurologist's work, although the possibility of organ donation now casts a shaft of sunlight on an otherwise sombre scene. Calixto Machado analyses three competing definitions of neurological death. He argues that consciousness is fundamental to the value we place on our lives but cautions against oversimple definitions of 'the place where consciousness dwells'.

AN INVITATION TO THE READER

The essays which follow have been written by contributors working around the world, with sharply differing backgrounds and perspectives. The essayists are united by an interest in the difficult ethical questions with which the practice of neurology confronts us daily. These are questions that may not have immediately conclusive answers: but we believe that some reflection on them provides valuable equipment with which to serve our patients better—whether one aspires to be a steely-nerved technician or a dog-eared wise physician.

REFERENCES

Antiplatelet Trialists' Collaboration (1994) Collaborative overview of randomised trials of antiplatelet therapy. 1. Prevention of death, myocardial infarction and stroke by prolonged antiplatelet therapy in various categories of patients. *British Medical Journal* **308**:81–106.

Bensimon G *et al.* (1994) A controlled trial of riluzole on amyotrophic lateral sclerosis. *New England Journal of Medicine* **330**:585–591.

Coney-Bloom J *et al.* (1998) A randomised trial evaluating the efficacy and safety of ENA 713 (rivastigmine tartrate), a new acetylcholinesterase inhibitor, in patients with mild to moderately severe Alzheimer's disease. *International Journal of Geriatric Psychopharmacology* **1**:55–65.

IFNB Multiple Sclerosis Study Group (1993) Interferon beta-1b is effective in relapsing-remitting multiple sclerosis-I: clinical results of a multicentre, randomised, double blind, placebo-controlled trial. *Neurology* **43**:655–661.

Rogers SI *et al.* (1998) A 24-week, double-blind, placebo-controlled trial of donepezil in patients with Alzheimer's disease. *Neurology* **50**:136–145.

1

What Are Ethics?

Anthony C Grayling

INTRODUCTION

When we think carefully about questions of how to live and to behave, and about whether certain of our choices and actions are right or wrong—in short, when we think carefully about our values—we are engaged in a characteristically philosophical activity, namely 'moral philosophy' or 'ethics'. When we wag our fingers at others and tell them what they should and should not do, we are engaged in a quite different activity, viz. moralizing. It might be expected, or at least hoped, that anyone who presumes to moralize does so on the basis of careful reflection on the principles underlying his strictures, and on the concepts (for example 'goodness', 'right', and 'duty') he employs. There is a tendency for some moralizers to rely on principles which were not acquired by the hard-won piecemeal method of critical reflection, but by the easy wholesale method of finding them ready-made among certain religious beliefs, or adopting them (whether as views or prejudices) from parents or contemporaries. Socrates famously remarked that 'the unexamined life is not worth living', meaning that the question of how to live and act is a serious one for each of us to consider with care. On this view, it is not enough to have a morality: one must have arrived at it, or at the very least accepted it, as a result of a conscious, deliberative process.

What applies to individuals applies to the communities they compose: every community has to debate with itself about the values and norms by which it defines itself. It scarcely needs saying that the need for such debate is now all the keener because, in addition to the moral dilemmas that humankind has always faced, dramatic new challenges are being posed by science—not least by medical science. This introduces a note of urgency into our deliberations. Humankind has progressed from making spears to making guided missiles, which does not alas suggest that we have made much moral progress in the same interval. Yet the rate of technological change is quickening exponentially: how are we to keep up if we do not think hard and clearly about what we want for human life and our world?

TWO PRELIMINARIES

This essay outlines the nature of ethical enquiry both in general and in particular application to medical practice. Two preliminaries need to be noted. One is that despite the apparent interchangeability of the expressions 'morals' and 'ethics', and of 'moral philosophy' and 'ethical enquiry (or reflection)', there is an important distinction between them. The term 'ethics' derives from a Greek root connoting personal character, whereas the term 'morals' derives from a Latin root connoting custom (compare the word 'mores'). Morality is standardly a matter of what is prescribed and proscribed in behaviour—what is permitted or forbidden—and therefore implies the apportionment of praise and blame, reward and punishment. It suggests the possibility of a code or of rules, a list consisting of injunctions which begin with phrases like 'thou shalt' and 'thou shalt not'. Ethics is a more inclusive notion, applying not just to certain kinds of conduct but to the whole character and quality of life. What colour you paint your house, and whether or not you cultivate musical and artistic tastes, might, on this view, be included in the topic of aesthetics, and in turn in the generally broader purview of ethical matters, but are not included among moral matters. Questions of ethics are therefore more comprehensive than those of morality. Of course, from the ethical choices one makes there flow actions (and inactions) which will be assessable for their more narrowly moral worth. Their ground will, however, lie not in moral rules but in the character of the life that produced them, and that makes a substantial difference.

The second preliminary is that we must observe a distinction between 'first order' and 'second order' questions. The first are those of practice, of what we are to do and refrain from doing. The Ten Commandments constitute a first order morality, because they enjoin us to behave in particular ways. When we take a step back and reflect upon the ideas and principles at work at the first order, we are engaged in a second order activity: we are not telling someone what to do, instead we are debating what justification there might be for telling someone that this or that is the 'right' thing to do or 'ought' or even 'must' be done. Second order questions are theoretical, first order questions are practical; at the second order we enquire into concepts, meanings, and reasons, while at the first order we give others or ourselves orders (or at least, recommendations).

THE DEVELOPMENT OF ETHICAL THEORY

As noted, ethics is the enquiry into how one should live. One good way to characterize it is to see what questions it attempts to answer. The two (related) questions that best identify its task are: what is 'goodness' (or, 'the good' or 'the good life') and, how ought one to act? Perhaps the sharpest way to define ethics is to see it as the attempt to answer the sceptic who cannot see why he should adjust his own actions, or compromise his own interests, in order to respect the interests and needs of others, and who therefore asks 'why bother to be moral?'.

As a systematic enquiry, ethics began in ancient Greece. Some of the Greek teachers of philosophy and rhetoric (collectively known as Sophists) argued that morality is a man-made convenience for the smoother running of society, and cannot therefore be binding; the rational course is therefore to pursue one's own interests. Plato responded that possession of virtues such as justice and courage promotes the good life, consisting of harmony in the soul. He makes his mouthpiece Socrates say that virtue is knowledge: if one knows the good, one cannot do wrong. His pupil Aristotle disagreed; one can indeed 'know the better but do the worse'—weakness of will is an all too human failing. Aristotle argued that the aim of life is happiness, which is achieved by acting in accordance with that faculty that uniquely defines mankind, namely reason. Reason teaches that the middle course in any situation is best; for example, courage is the mean between cowardice and rashness, generosity is the mean between meanness and profligacy. The man of practical wisdom will always determine the mean in any situation, and act accordingly. If you find that you are not much good at making such judgements, you need only emulate the man of practical wisdom.

Not everyone found Aristotle's middle way (middle aged, middle class?) view convincing. Chief among the later Greek schools were the Epicureans and Stoics. Epicurus held that pleasure is the highest good, by 'pleasure' meaning friendship and conversation. Love, sex, drinking and feasting, he austerely remarked, carry the seeds of pain, so they must be avoided. The Stoics taught indifference; what we cannot control we must accept, and what we can control—our own private passions and desires—we must subdue. In this way we liberate ourselves to live simply and 'in accordance with nature'. The two great teachers of Stoicism occupied the opposite ends of the scale: they were Epictetus, who was a Greek slave in a Roman household, and Marcus Aurelius, who was a Roman emperor. Stoicism was the dominating outlook of educated people in Hellenic and Roman antiquity for five hundred years. In the end it was superseded by Christianity, a belief system that did not brook competitors. Stoicism gave us the colloquial senses of 'stoical' and 'philosophical' we are familiar with today, as in 'he was very ill, but he put up with it philosophically'.

Ethical thought changed character dramatically under Christianity. Belief in a divine lawgiver removes the need to enquire into the source and justification of ethical laws. But the great Christian moral philosophers, Augustine and Thomas Aquinas, nevertheless, tried to marry Greek philosophy to Christian moral teaching. Under Aristotle's influence, Aquinas analysed human acts as those we have a reason to perform, the reason ultimately being to achieve happiness, which we do by fulfilling human purposes according to God-ordained natural laws.

Most Christian morality, however, took the form of casuistry, the careful interpretation of prohibitions and permissions (when must one fast? who among my relatives can I marry?). But even in this guise it faces difficulties. Is the Good good because God commands it, or does he command it because it is good? This question reveals the weakness of theological ethics. If the former, then ethics is based on arbitrary will, and we have no better reason to obey it than if someone coerces us by threats to do such-and-such. This is indeed, how, religious ethics works: it promises or threatens, respectively, ultimate—indeed, eternal—rewards or punishments. If the latter, there must be some independent source of value.

Accordingly, the philosophers of the early modern period returned to basics, to an examination of underlying principles. Does morality arise from love of others, or of self? Is it the child of reason, or of emotion? Thomas Hobbes argued, as some of the Sophists had done, that morality stems from self-interest. In the state of nature self-interest produces conflicts, so men gather into society, contracting to forego some personal liberty for mutual advantage. But this contract, in turn, requires an absolute sovereign to ensure its enforcement. In opposition to Hobbes's egoism, Butler and Shaftesbury argued that people are by nature altruistic, seeking the public good as well as their own. They thus offered benevolence as the basis of morality. In this they found an ally in David Hume, for whom the basis of morality is human sentiment, and in particular sympathy. Hume thought that the only motive anyone could have for performing any action is emotion; he found it impossible to believe that cold reason by itself could spur one to act one way or another, or at all. In sharp contrast, Immanuel Kant accorded reason this very role. To act morally, he says, we must act according to those principles which reason identifies as everywhere applicable; universalizable statements of duty constitute the moral law, and the 'good will' is that which seeks always to do its duty.

The revived debate about morality's principles did not seem to Jeremy Bentham and John Stuart Mill to offer a simple and practical moral theory that the man in the street could apply. They therefore developed Frances Hutcheson's 'utilitarian' suggestion that those actions are good which promote 'the greatest happiness of the greatest number', and offered this as an effective rule to help people decide how to act. Their view rapidly secured a hold on Anglo-Saxon minds, and formed the outlook of generations of young men who went abroad as British imperial administrators. But even as it did so, a radically different challenge was being formulated elsewhere: Friedrich Nietzsche attacked Christian ethics as a 'slave morality' because it turned the negative experiences of exiled Israel—its suffering, poverty and enslavement—into the virtues of the Beatitudes: 'blessed are the meek … blessed are they that mourn'. In its place Nietzsche urged the opposite: the morality of the superman, the higher kind of individual we should all aspire to be by living lofty lives that overcome the conformism and barbarism that always threatens to engulf us.

Ethical debate in the earlier twentieth century expresses frustration with the effort to base morality on a given set of principles. G. E. Moore claimed that the concept of goodness is indefinable, that we (or at least some of us) have a faculty of moral sense by which we can simply 'intuit' the presence of goodness in persons or their actions, and that the chief goods are friendship and beauty.

(A familiar joke about the members of the Bloomsbury Group, who were much influenced by Moore, is that they practised moral economy by having beautiful friends.) The Logical Positivists held that moral assertions are strictly speaking meaningless because they are not the kind of assertion that can be evaluated for truth or falsity; at most they have only exhortatory or persuasive uses. Some have harkened back to Hobbes and others have based morality in self-interest. John Mackie defended an 'enlightened' version of such a thesis by saying that self-interest makes people behave well towards their fellows because they rationally grasp that it benefits themselves to do so.

Such views seem to suggest that morality rests upon a less than absolute foundation. Perhaps relativism is true: what one person or group takes to be right is taken to be wrong by another person or group, and there is no way of deciding between them. Perhaps morality is entirely a matter of current preferences in society: 'nothing is good or bad but thinking makes it so'. There are of course those who continue to argue vigorously that there are moral truths, and that truth is independent of what we humans like and dislike. Someone who thinks in these terms is a 'moral objectivist' or 'moral realist'. Relativism is one form of 'moral anti-realism', but not the only form, for there are those who argue that our morality stems from facts about us and our preferences, but these facts and preferences find universal expression among human beings, as rational reflection shows; and that therefore bald confrontation of contradictory values is not irresolvable.

What this summary of the history of ethical debate shows is that questions about the nature of moral value, and those about the grounds of moral choice and action, are delicate and vexed. Yet ethical questions are practical ones: we are all frequently faced with ethical choices, some of them extremely difficult, and we feel the want of guidelines. In the case where our technological abilities far outrun any consensus about what is right or good in the cases they apply to, we are in an urgent dilemma. This is especially so in medicine.

MEDICINE AND ETHICS

Some writers on medical ethics note that until quite recently the two ethical injunctions by which medical people lived were: do not advertise, and do not have sexual relations with your patients. There was of course an adherence, at least implicitly, to the professional code suggested by the Hippocratic ideal of confidentiality, cure where possible but avoidance of harm at least, and always care. In that ideal the focus of attention is the relationship between the practitioner and his patient; that of course remains so in the much more extensive set of considerations which now constitute medical ethics. In these the questions about the practitioner–patient relationship are more complex and diverse. They concern patients' rights, their consent to treatment, the practitioner's duty to tell patients the truth, the degree to which paternalism is justified, and how the practitioner is to decide in cases of divided loyalties—as when public health considerations arise, or when a patient would be suitable as an experimental subject in testing an important new treatment. From the beginning of life to its end—from abortion and withholding treatment from severely deformed neonates, to difficulties about providing the elderly with life-sustaining treatment, and on to euthanasia—ethical dilemmas multiply and press.

The ethical nightmares of contemporary technologized medicine were first prompted by the introduction of life-support systems and kidney dialysis machines. Given that the number of dialysis machines was, in the early days, far outstripped by the number of patients needing them, committees had to be established to choose who would receive treatment. That difficult task was made harder by the result of early studies showing that the patients chosen for treatment tended to resemble the committee members themselves in respect of social and educational profile. Life-support technology introduced a now distressingly familiar related dilemma. As the much-publicized case of Karen Quinlan in the early 1970s showed, the question of when life-support should be ended for patients in a persistent vegetative state, and of who has the right to decide, is hard to answer and still sometimes has to be settled on a case-by-case basis in courts of law.

Indeed the medical profession finds itself confronted by thorny problems on almost every front. In paediatrics, neurology and psychiatry, practitioners find themselves dealing with patients who are not competent to contribute to decisions about their own treatment. In all aspects of reproductive medicine there are familiar but very hard choices about fertility, surrogacy, parenthood, the fate and rights of possible future persons, and much besides. In every general practitioner's surgery, limitation of resources means rationing, entailing choices about who will get treated, and who not, and for what, and why. The demand on busy general practitioners to make these difficult decisions is hard enough on them; it is harder still on patients, whose chances of treatment, even of survival, therefore become a lottery.

All the problems mentioned have the gritty feel of real-life difficulties which readers of these pages will either have encountered in one or another variant, or at any rate will recognize as part of the atmosphere of concern in contemporary medicine. But behind them lie other questions, in one sense abstractly philosophical, but in another acutely close to the practical difficulties experienced on wards and in consulting rooms. Some of them might at first glance seem to be entirely practical, but a moment's reflection reveals their underlying conceptual content. Among them are the following: What is a person? What do we mean by 'rights' when we accord persons rights? Is a fetus a person? If not, does a fetus have rights anyway? Is a frozen embryo a person? When does life begin? When does it end? How does one define 'benefit' and 'harm'? When does something count as a 'treatment'? Are doctors always obliged to help their patients? Must doctors always save life? Is it not sometimes justified and humane to end life rather than to prolong it? Are young people more valuable and therefore more entitled to treatment than old or older people? What is the definition of a 'worthwhile life'? Is a person with a family more valuable than one without? Should one never experiment on embryos? Does a woman have an exclusive and total right to determine what happens in and to her body, including the right to choose continuation or termination of pregnancy? If a treatment for a given condition exists, does everyone with that condition have a right to such treatment? Who decides what treatment shall be given to individuals (such as those with dementia) who are without representatives or competence to share in decision-making?

One could extend the list, but its purport is already clear. There are few sharp definitions, and few easy answers, in connection with the intimate, often invasive, vexed, and unequal relationship between the knowledge-and-technology possessing doctor and his or her vulnerable, perhaps afraid, and usually less well informed patient. Medicine is one of the places where the dilemmas of ethics present themselves most acutely, for these reasons. It is fortunate that many of those who choose to work in medicine are, by inclination, among the best equipped to think them through with intelligence, generosity, and compassion.

It should be clear, also, that *medical ethics* are appropriately named. They bear on the totality of the relationship between doctor and patient—an exceptionally sensitive relationship which turns on conceptions of human nature, rights, interests and responsibilities and which can affect the entire quality and character of the lives of those involved.

AN EXAMPLE DEBATE: PATERNALISM AND THE AUTONOMY OF THE PATIENT

A central and characteristic example of ethical dilemmas in medicine is the case where the patient is not able to share in decisions about treatment, and where therefore the practitioner seems to have a duty to make the decision on his or her behalf.

We might aspire, in ethically ideal circumstances, to accord respect to each individual we encounter (at least until he forfeits it in a way that genuinely merits forfeiture) and correlatively to treat each individual as autonomous, that is, as being in charge of his own life (as shown by the etymology of the term, it connotes the state of being a lawgiver to oneself: the antonym is 'heteronymous'). Of course, there are so many social, legal, moral and psychological constraints on true autonomy for each of us, owing in part to our membership of society and in part to the finite character of our intellects and experience, that the concept of autonomy is an idealization. But the ethical goal is for each individual to have the maximum degree of autonomy consistent with these social and natural restrictions.

The notions of autonomy and respect are asymmetrically linked. We respect the needs, interests and concerns of a young child even though we do not think he is autonomous, or fully autonomous. We recognize that autonomous agents might, by virtue of their independently chosen actions, forfeit respect. But it is a principal part of according respect to individuals that we treat them as autonomous. When in some way we cease to treat them so, we are being what has aptly been called 'paternalistic'—as implied by the heteronymity of children, which justifies us in acting on their behalf, taking decisions for them and directing their lives in what we judge to be their interests, for so long as they are incompetent to choose for themselves because they are insufficiently equipped with experience, knowledge and powers of mind.

It is a familiar fact that medical practitioners are especially apt to feel the tension between respecting autonomy and being justifiably paternalistic. Few patients, however intelligent and informed otherwise, can really be held to know enough about their condition and its available treatments to be full partners in decisions about what should best be done. Sometimes patients are unconscious and cannot take any part in making those decisions. When a practitioner knows what is in a patient's interests, but the patient refuses to take the treatment advised, is he ever justified in administering the treatment nonetheless?

One class of cases can immediately be left aside: those that involve third parties. If a patient is carrying a serious communicable disease, the interests of third parties are at stake and a patient can justifiably be required to accept treatment for the disease, or at least be prevented from spreading it. This degree of paternalism was accepted by John Stuart Mill, who otherwise was strongly of the view that:

> the sole end for which mankind are warranted, individually or collectively, in interfering with the liberty of action of any of their number is self-protection ... the only purpose for which power can be rightfully exercised over any member of a civilized community, against his will, is ... to prevent harm to others. His own good, either physical or moral, is not a sufficient warrant.

A powerful argument supports this liberal tenet. It is that if one granted that a given body such as the state were licensed to decide what is in others' interest, there would be no obvious limit to the authority it could exercise over them. As Isaiah Berlin put it, it could 'bully, oppress, torture them in the name, and on behalf, of their "real" selves, in the secure knowledge that whatever is the true goal of man (happiness, performance of duty, wisdom, a just society, self-fulfilment) must be identical with his freedom—the free choice of his "true", albeit often submerged and inarticulate, self'.

Mill also of course allowed paternalism in the case of children and the mentally impaired, but—much more riskily, from the viewpoint of his principles—he conceded that it would be justified to stop a man from walking onto a bridge which he did not know was in a dangerous condition. This concession is exactly one that a medical practitioner might appeal to in the case of a patient who does not or seems not to grasp the seriousness of his condition and the advisability of a given treatment. He might also do it on the basis of an argument to the conclusion that sometimes a paternalistic authority better knows not just what an individual's interests are, but what his preferences would be if he were properly informed or able to judge.

It has for example been argued that a competent official could well 'respect your own preferences better than you would have done through your actions'. Take the case of tobacco smoking: a superficial preference to smoke cigarettes conflicts with a deeper preference to stay alive and well. The latter is not only a deeper but a more settled and relevant preference than the former. Consider a young person who smokes because he wishes to appear sophisticated, or to conform to the behaviour of his peers; on this view an appropriate authority would be justified in preventing him on the grounds that he will, in time, himself come to a stable view that smoking is harmful. He is currently distracted and misinformed about his real interests, and is therefore not able to protect them. This applies even more to a medical patient choosing or acting in ways inimical to his interests.

Even if one rejected the 'slippery slope' argument that underlies Isaiah Berlin's view, however, one could say that autonomy is such a crucial value that even the clearest case of a patient's choosing or acting in direct opposition to his interests cannot justify a doctor in overriding his decision and acting against his wishes. Of course, where a patient is demented, comatose, or otherwise mentally incapacitated, and has no competent family to decide, a responsible doctor or hospital ethics committee can and must do it for him. But the envisaged case is one where an ordinarily rational person, even if not able to understand every intricacy of his condition and the treatment options, rejects his practitioners advice; and where only he is going to be affected by his decision. On this view, even if he pulls out his intravenous lines and walks out of the hospital, with the medical staff knowing that he is likely to die within hours, he has to be allowed to act as he chooses. Is such a view tenable, in the face of the practitioners' duties and vocation, and their belief that he might, if he let them help him recover, be grateful that they restrained him after all?

Principles of autonomy and liberty here conflict with paternalism in cases—one could convincingly and almost endlessly multiply them—where some form or degree of the latter appears reasonable and justifiable. This is a crucial problem because proposed solutions (or compromises) affect almost everything else in medical ethics, which concerns not only personhood, consent, the aims of medical intervention, and even decisions about the quality of life that medical interventions can offer, but also raises questions about the duties and rights of medical practitioners, which is to say the very point of their vocation. This is illustrated by what might at first seem a marginal consideration. In the sketch just given I have omitted considerations about the therapeutic value of the practitioner's assumption of authority and the confidence this can generate in some patients. Before the advent of technologized and biochemicalized medicine, this and regimen were the physician's principal tools. Perhaps the psychological power once inherent in certified possession of theoretical and practical knowledge counts for much less now; we live in a dispensation where professional authority and the paternalism it once both licensed and required is no longer what it was. Certainly, in the face of growing assertions of autonomy and individual liberty, paternalism is regarded as intrinsically wrong unless it is well fortified by arguments tailored to specific cases. In this way questions about autonomy and paternalism affect the fundamentals of the doctor–patient relationship, and lie at the heart of the ethical dimension of medicine.

CONCLUDING REMARKS

Ethical dilemmas in medicine assume different guises, depending on circumstances, just as the problem of paternalism does. That is a function of the variety of human interests and concerns, and the way that context renders them unique. It does not follow that it is wrong to seek general principles in ethics, for at the very least principles can serve as a starting point, a guide, or a touchstone, in finding ways of dealing with specific problems. Ethical reflection does not promise solutions that are invariably, or even very often, neat or satisfying; most of the time they are likely to be the opposite, ending as messy compromises, or as the least bad among a set of unpromising alternatives, despite all the thought and negotiation we can manage. But that is how it is in human affairs, which gives us all the more reason to try to think clearly about questions of principle when we have opportunities to do so: not in the rush of the emergency room or operating theatre, but in the spaces we give ourselves for study and thought. The point is to be prepared—if not with answers, then at the very least with a clear awareness of the kinds of questions we are likely to face, and with some sense of the answers, even if they are competing answers, that others have offered.

BIBLIOGRAPHY

Bell JM and Mendus S (1988) *Philosophy and Medical Welfare*. Cambridge: Cambridge University Press.
Brock D (1993) *Life and Death*. Cambridge: Cambridge University Press.
Buchanan A and Brock D (1990) *Deciding for Others*. Cambridge: Cambridge University Press.
Gillon R and Lloyd A (1994) *Principles of Health Care Ethics*. New York: John Wiley and Sons.
Glover J (1977) *Causing Death and Saving Lives*. London: Penguin.
Harris J (1985) *The Value of Life*. London: Routledge.
Lockwood M (1985) *Moral Dilemmas in Modern Medicine*. Oxford: Oxford University Press.

Diagnosis and communication

2

Should Consent Be Required for an HIV Test?

Rebecca Dresser

ABSTRACT

In the years since the emergence of the HIV/AIDS epidemic, some clinicians and other writers have argued for the adoption of compulsory HIV testing policies. Such policies would depart from the general rule that patients should make their own decisions on whether to accept the physical and social risks of a medical procedure. Moreover, a close look at the potential consequences of mandatory testing in the general population suggests that its benefit would not outweigh its ethical and financial costs. Mandatory testing has also been endorsed for selected populations, including hospitalized patients, clinicians, pregnant women, infants and immigrants. In each situation, however, the justification for such testing is questionable.

INTRODUCTION

During the 1980s, scientists developed blood tests to detect persons infected with the human immunodeficiency virus (HIV). With the availability of clinical testing came strong debate over its appropriate application. Initially, a few writers advocated universal compulsory testing, together with quarantine or other coercive measures aimed at containing the infection (Buckley, 1986; Fallone, 1988). Most analysts, however, argued that individual consent should be a prerequisite to HIV testing, except in selected situations presenting unusually strong justification for imposed testing (Bayer *et al.*, 1986; Swartz 1988; Lo *et al.*, 1989). Existing ethical and policy recommendations incorporate the latter approach (Quinn 1992; CDC 1993), although empirical research suggests that these recommendations are not always observed in practice (Lewis and Montgomery, 1990; Pomeroy *et al.*, 1994).

HIV TESTING IN THE GENERAL POPULATION

Advocates of a requirement for individual consent to HIV testing present several reasons for their position. First, they invoke general moral and legal principles assigning significance to the individual's interests in making decisions affecting his or her physical integrity, health care, and overall well-being. Individuals deciding whether to undergo a medical procedure typically consider its risks and potential benefits, and any available alternative courses of action. Their ultimate decisions reflect their particular values and circumstances, and sometimes depart from what health care professionals see as the advisable choice.

The HIV test's risks, potential benefits, and alternatives depend on a specific individual's personal and social situation. Persons with symptoms of infection usually will accept testing because the results can be relevant to the selection of an appropriate treatment regimen. Until recently, however, asymptomatic individuals could obtain few clinical benefits from learning their HIV status. On the other hand, a positive HIV test result can adversely affect a person's employment and health insurance status, and have other negative effects on a person's life. Attempts to maintain confidentiality frequently are unsuccessful, and test results may become known to a variety of persons. For some patients, then, the medical benefit of early testing may be outweighed by its detrimental consequences (Gunderson *et al.*, 1996). The moral principle of respect for persons supports giving individuals the authority to make their own choices on whether to expose themselves to the adverse consequences of testing (Bayer *et al.*, 1986; Lo *et al.*, 1989). The potential social costs associated with a positive HIV test have led many state government officials to establish more stringent consent requirements for this test than are normally required in the context of diagnostic testing (Gostin and Webber, 1998).

Although the individual's interest in making important personal decisions merits strong respect, it is sometimes defensible to override that interest to advance other morally significant considerations. In the context of HIV testing, the primary competing consideration is the goal of preventing other persons from becoming infected. Proponents of compulsory testing argue that 'once they are identified by a test, infected persons can prevent new infections by discontinuing behavior that spreads the virus' (Weiss and Thier, 1988).

Yet many others contend that voluntary testing is the most reasonable and cost-effective method of protecting others. A universal compulsory testing programme would be extremely expensive to administer. Such a programme would be much broader in scope than any existing health screening programme, and would require everyone to be tested periodically to detect new cases of infection (Bayer *et al.*, 1986). Proponents of voluntary testing also note that testing itself cannot prevent the spread of disease. Persons found to be infected must then choose or be forced to behave in ways that remove or minimize the chance of transmitting the infection to others. Because massive quarantine and other coercive measures to contain and label infected persons would be morally unacceptable, as well as highly impractical, voluntary behaviour change is the desired outcome of testing. This outcome is more likely to occur in a supportive programme in which tests are performed for persons who consent to the procedure after a discussion of its risks and anticipated benefits. Many analysts also believe that protection of persons in the general population can be achieved through widespread public education on behavioural strategies for minimizing virus exposure (Bayer *et al.*, 1986).

In sum, the most ethical and practically attainable method of advancing the interests of others in avoiding infection is to implement supportive programmes requiring informed consent to HIV testing, as well as public instruction on ways individuals can reduce their risk of exposure (Bayer *et al.*, 1986; Weiss and Thier, 1988). Contemporary discussion of the ethics of HIV testing focuses on the challenge of implementing a workable and cost-effective system offering testing and counselling to a large number of potentially infected persons (De Cock and Johnson, 1998).

The US Centers for Disease Control (CDC) recommend that hospitals with relatively high rates of HIV-infected patients offer voluntary testing and counselling services to all patients aged 15–54 with a primary diagnosis other than HIV or acquired immune deficiency disorder (CDC, 1993). Financially strapped hospitals face significant difficulties in complying with these recommendations, however, and implementation rates are believed to be quite low (Gunderson *et al.*, 1996). A recent proposal which attempts to balance cost considerations and ethical principles suggests that all patients in the target population be provided upon admission or registration 'written information about HIV and the HIV test, a statement that someone will ask permission for an HIV test—typically while conducting a routine blood draw—and ... a phone number to call for more information or to withdraw consent within 48 hours' (Gunderson *et al.*, 1996).

HIV TESTING IN THE CLINICAL SETTING

Though voluntary testing is the preferred approach in the general population, there is stronger support for mandatory testing in certain circumstances in which the test's benefits to others are more clear. For example, mandatory testing of all blood, semen, and organ donors is widely accepted. In these situations, testing offers a highly effective means of protecting recipients from infection. At the same time, blood, semen, and organ donation programmes can respect the individual's freedom to decide whether to undergo HIV testing by informing prospective donors that they will be tested and allowing them to withdraw if they prefer to avoid the procedure (Bayer *et al.*, 1986).

Mandatory testing for other groups is more controversial. Most relevant to clinicians are proposals for routine mandatory testing of (1) hospitalized persons; (2) clinicians involved in surgery or other invasive procedures on patients; and (3) pregnant women and newborns.

Physicians and others favouring mandatory testing of hospital patients argue that clinicians ought to be given the opportunity to detect an HIV-positive patient so that they can take special precautions to avoid exposure to blood and other potentially infectious body fluids. Some writers support the incorporation of HIV tests into the array of procedures routinely performed on hospitalized patients without prior discussion of the risks, potential benefits and other information relevant to each procedure (Brandt *et al.*, 1990). Others seek to make HIV testing a condition of acceptance for clinical care. For example, some surgeons claim a right to require HIV testing and to refuse to operate on HIV-positive persons: 'I look forward to the availability of routine screening of surgical patients for HIV and reserve the right to decline to operate on those in whom recent or continuing infection with HIV is likely other than in lifethreatening circumstances' (Guy, 1987).

Opponents of these proposals offer several arguments in defence of their view. First, standard HIV tests cannot detect infected persons who have not yet developed antibodies to HIV. Thus, this form of testing is not an accurate way to detect all patients with the potential to transmit infection to clinicians. A negative antibody test can induce 'a false sense of security and could possibly increase the occupational risks' to clinicians taking fewer precautions with such patients (Brandt *et al.*, 1990). Newer diagnostic tests identifying viral antigens allow more accuracy in detecting infection, but these tests are not always available (Gostin *et al.*, 1994). More importantly, CDC officials note that available 'information does not support the belief that knowledge of a patient's HIV status decreases the risk of infection for health care workers' by leading them to exercise greater caution (CDC, 1993). Health care workers can more effectively protect themselves from HIV (and other viral infections such as hepatitis) by treating all patients as potentially infectious. This realization underlies the *Universal Blood and Body Fluid Precautions* now recommended for clinicians in all health care settings (CDC, 1988). Transmission risks could be further reduced through research on methods to lessen the rate of needle-sticks and surgical exposures (Brandt *et al.*, 1990).

Second, testing without a patient's awareness or permission departs from the informed consent principles normally applicable in the health care setting. Though HIV testing poses minimal physical risk to patients, the psychological and social risks are sufficiently high to distinguish this test from more routine diagnostic testing. One physician relayed the following poignant example:

> In 1985, I was the primary physician for a young man whose life was ruined by the inappropriate disclosure of a positive human immunodeficiency virus (HIV)-antibody test. A physician ordered the test without consent and notified the local health department of the positive result. The health department notified the individual's employer and he was promptly fired. These events became common knowledge at his workplace and in his rural Midwestern town and he was shunned. His landlord asked him to move. Ten days after testing, the life he had known for the past ten years was permanently ruined and he left town. With the loss of his job came loss of health insurance and insurability; he has been unable to obtain health or life insurance since then. (Sherer, 1988)

Besides the potential harm to infected individuals from unwanted HIV testing, such testing could have adverse public health consequences. This is because 'failure to assure patients that informed consent will be respected in clinical or hospital settings is likely to lead those individuals most likely to be infected to avoid settings in which they may be tested without their knowledge and consent' (Brandt *et al.*, 1990). Concerned individuals will be more willing to obtain HIV testing if they perceive the clinical setting as a place in which their desires for information and control are respected rather than disregarded by clinicians engaged in secret or compulsory testing.

A narrower version of the proposal for compelled testing of persons receiving clinical care is to mandate testing when a clinician receives an accidental needle-stick injury. Some states currently authorize such testing (Gostin and Webber, 1998). Coerced testing is usually unnecessary, for most patients will consent to an HIV test if a needle-stick injury occurs. There is growing evidence that postexposure chemoprophylaxis can effectively prevent infection, though the treatment carries health risks as well (Henderson, 1997). If HIV antigen tests become widely available, the pressure for mandatory testing in this context is likely to increase, given that individuals with possible exposure will seek to determine whether the risks of undergoing chemoprophylaxis are outweighed by the risk of HIV infection.

Many organizations and commentators dispute the claim that physicians have a right to condition care on a patient's willingness to undergo testing. Most respond that such a right would unacceptably conflict with the traditional role and ethical responsibilities of physicians. Physicians understandably seek to avoid becoming infected; some also express their 'reluctance to expose ... their staff, and families to the risk of contracting this terrible disease' (Guy, 1987). But many physicians and others contend that considerations of social justice and professional obligation support rules requiring physicians to accept the very small health risks accompanying the care of HIV-positive patients. This view is adopted in the following American Medical Association statement: '[a] physician may not ethically refuse to treat a patient whose condition is within the physician's current realm of competence solely because the patient is seropositive for HIV' (Council on Ethical and Judicial Affairs, 1994). Some surgeons and other physicians dissent from this view, but it appears that the vast majority of clinicians are willing to accept the small health risks accompanying care of persons with HIV (Peterson, 1989).

Also controversial are proposals for mandatory testing of clinicians to protect their patients from infection. US federal law requires states to follow Centers for Disease Control guidelines, which advise testing for clinicians performing certain invasive procedures deemed to present the greatest risk of HIV and hepatitis transmission to patients. The guidelines further state that infected clinicians should seek expert advice on whether the procedures can be performed safely and should alert patients to their infectious status before undertaking such procedures (CDC, 1991). American Medical Association policy states that physicians who know they are HIV positive 'should consult colleagues as to which activities the physician can pursue without creating a risk to patients' (Council on Ethical and Judicial Affairs, 1994).

Some writers contend that this voluntary testing policy is inadequate, and endorse instead mandatory clinician testing and mandatory practice restrictions on infected clinicians. But others note the extremely low risk of clinician–patient transmission and the high expense of operating an ongoing testing programme. They also express concern that mandatory clinician testing could reduce clinicians' willingness to accept the risks entailed in treating persons who are HIV positive. In the light of these considerations, the preferred method of avoiding clinician–patient transmission is to combine voluntary testing programmes with efforts to eliminate transmission risks through modifying traditional surgical and other invasive techniques (Gerberding, 1996). At the same time, some state courts have ruled that HIV-positive clinicians have a legal duty to disclose this information to patients or public health officials (Gostin and Webber, 1998).

Mandatory testing of pregnant women or infants has also attracted some support. Testing pregnant women can reduce the incidence of maternal–infant transmission. Some infected women will choose pregnancy termination. Others will accept antiretroviral treatment that significantly reduces the incidence of infection in infants (Goldstein and Sever, 1996). Testing infants themselves can allow physicians to provide enhanced medical care to HIV-positive infants. Mandatory testing in either form involves mandatory testing of women, however, because an infant's positive test definitively indicates that the mother is infected.

Opponents of mandatory testing for pregnant women or infants question the justification for such testing. They predict that this approach will deter some women from seeking prenatal and other medical care, which will in turn have a detrimental impact on their own and their infants' health (Simonds *et al.*, 1996). They also note that when women are informed of the availability of testing and its therapeutic rationale, a substantial percentage consent to HIV tests for themselves or their infants (Limata *et al.*, 1997). For these reasons, the CDC continue to recommend voluntary testing in this context (CDC, 1995). In 1996, however, the state of New York enacted legislation authorizing mandatory HIV testing of infants and mandatory disclosure of test results to parents (McKinney's, 1997). Although some clinicians welcomed this development, others argued that if protecting infant health is deemed to justify compulsory HIV testing, such testing should be conducted directly on pregnant women. Infants would benefit much more from such a programme, they contended, because pregnant women testing positive could then be offered immediate treatment with the potential to prevent infection in many of the infants born to such women (Sontag, 1997). This view did not prevail, however, probably because officials wanted to avoid physical coercion of adult women and the potential deterrent effect of imposed testing on prenatal care.

HIV TESTING IN OTHER CONTEXTS

Mandatory testing is endorsed in other selected situations. For example, mandatory testing of criminal defendants is defended in cases of possible HIV transmission to sexual assault victims (Gostin *et al.*, 1994). Two states adopted, then discontinued, mandatory premarital HIV testing when it was found that the programmes detected few cases at great cost and also reduced the number of marriages in those states (Wilkerson, 1989).

Persons in the military, immigrants, prisoners, and intravenous drug users have also been subjected to mandatory HIV testing (Dickens, 1990). The justification for each type of mandatory testing programme varies. A particular target of criticism is US immigration policy, which gives officials discretion to impose HIV testing on temporary visitors and requires such testing for permanent residence applicants (whose applications are denied if they test positive). Critics contend that the programme is unjust and encourages travellers and immigrants to falsify their HIV status or to avoid the authorities altogether by staying underground (Gostin *et al.*, 1990). Health and life insurance companies also may require individual applicants to undergo HIV testing for underwriting purposes (Jarvis *et al.*, 1991). The practice of using such tests as the basis to exclude persons from health insurance coverage raises general questions on public and private sector responsibilities to ensure that adequate health care is available to persons in need.

CONCLUSION

The predominant view is that strong moral and practical justification exists for adopting informed patient consent as a prerequisite to HIV testing. With few exceptions, the consensus is that persons should be free to determine for themselves whether to accept the potential burdens associated with testing, in order to obtain its therapeutic and other potential benefits. Most analysts believe that the societal goal of minimizing disease transmission can be achieved through voluntary testing combined with measures such as universal precautions, refinements in surgical and other invasive procedures, and promotion of 'safe sex' and other preventive measures among the general public.

Advances in antiretroviral therapy for HIV infection could also reduce the support for mandatory testing programmes. In the future, pressures for involuntary testing are likely to diminish if the number of persons willing to undergo testing increases. With the development of more effective treatment options, more individuals are likely to perceive a clear personal benefit to HIV testing, and to seek testing voluntarily (Brandt *et al.*, 1990). If scientists are successful in developing an HIV vaccine, uninfected persons will gain an additional opportunity to protect themselves from infection.

The rate of voluntary testing is also likely to increase if the detrimental effects of HIV testing are reduced. Although a positive HIV diagnosis will inevitably be accompanied by psychological burdens, clinicians and policymakers can work to lessen its adverse effects on the individual's employment and insurance status, and to reduce other forms of discrimination against persons infected with HIV.

Today, the greatest ethical and policy challenge is to implement effective voluntary testing programmes. Testing programmes must supply the information, counselling, and clinical support that can encourage infected individuals to act in ways that minimize the chances of transmission to others (Limata *et al.*, 1997). Clinicians would be well advised to focus their efforts on creating and conducting such programmes. High-quality voluntary testing programmes, better therapies, and a more accepting social climate for persons testing positive are the preferred approaches to achieving the ultimate goals of delivering treatment and other assistance to affected individuals and minimizing the spread of HIV infection. For now, clinicians faced with HIV testing issues should consider the following general guidelines: (1) offer HIV testing to all at-risk individuals; (2) promote voluntary HIV testing programmes that include prior disclosure of risks and potential benefits as well as post-test counselling; (3) observe reasonable precautions to avoid viral transmission in the health care setting; and (4) offer high-quality health care to seropositive individuals.

REFERENCES

Bayer R, Levine C and Wolf SM (1986) HIV antibody screening: an ethical framework for evaluating proposed programs. *Journal of the American Medical Association* **256**:1768–1774.
Brandt AM, Cleary PD and Gostin LO (1990) Routine hospital testing for HIV: an ethical and legal challenge. In: *AIDS and the Health Care System* (ed. LO Gostin), pp. 125–139. New Haven: Yale University.
Buckley WF (1986) Combating the AIDS epidemic: identify all the carriers. *New York Times*, March 18.
CDC (1988) Update: universal precautions for prevention of transmission of human immunodeficiency virus, hepatitis B virus, and other bloodborne pathogens in health-care settings. *MMWR* **24**:377–388.
CDC (1991) Recommendations for preventing transmission of human immunodeficiency virus and hepatitis B virus to patients during exposure-prone invasive procedures. *MMWR* **40**:1–9.
CDC (1993) Recommendations for HIV testing services for inpatients and outpatients in acute-care hospital settings. *MMWR* **42**:1–6.
CDC (1995) US Public Health Service recommendations for human immunodeficiency virus counseling and voluntary testing for pregnant women. *MMWR* **44**:1–15.
Council on Ethical and Judicial Affairs, American Medical Association (1994) *Code of Medical Ethics: Current Opinions with Annotations*, p. 145. Chicago: American Medical Association.
De Cock KM and Johnson AM (1998) From exceptionalism to normalisation: a reappraisal of attitudes and practice around HIV testing. *British Medical Journal* **316**:290–293.
Dickens BM (1990) Confidentiality and the duty to warn. In: *AIDS and the Health Care System* (ed LO Gostin), pp. 98–112. New Haven: Yale University.
Fallone EA (1988) Preserving the public health: a proposal to quarantine recalcitrant AIDS carriers. *Boston University Law Review* **68**:441–505.
Gerberding JL (1996) The infected health care provider. *New England Journal of Medicine* **334**:594–595.
Goldstein PJ and Sever J (1996) Preventing perinatal HIV transmission. *Journal of the American Medical Association* **276**:779.
Gostin LO, Cleary PD, Mayer KH *et al.* (1990) Screening immigrants and international travelers for the human immunodeficiency virus. *New England Journal of Medicine* **322**:1743–1746.
Gostin LO, Lazzarini Z, Alexander D *et al* (1994) HIV testing, counseling, and prophylaxis after sexual assault. *Journal of the American Medical Association* **271**:1436–1444.

Gostin LO and Webber DW. (1998) HIV infection and AIDS in the public health and health care systems. *Journal of the American Medical Association* **279**:1108–1113.

Gunderson M, Mayo D and Rhame F (1996) Routine HIV testing of hospital patients and pregnant women: informed consent in the real world. *Kennedy Institute of Ethics Journal* **6**:161–182.

Guy PJ (1987) AIDS: a doctor's duty. *British Medical Journal* **294**:445.

Henderson DK (1997) Postexposure treatment of HIV—taking some risks for safety's sake. *New England Journal of Medicine* **337**:1542–1543.

Jarvis RM, Closen ML, Hermann DHJ *et al.* (1991) *AIDS Law*, pp. 134–142. St Paul, Minn: West.

Lewis CE and Montgomery K (1990) The HIV-testing policies of US hospitals. *Journal of the American Medical Association* **264**:2764–2767.

Limata C, Schoen EJ and Cohen D (1997) Compliance with voluntary prenatal HIV testing in a large health maintenance organization. *Journal of Acquired Immune Deficiency Syndromes and Human Retrovirology* **15**:126–130.

Lo B, Steinbrook RL, Cooke M *et al.* (1989) Voluntary screening for human immunodeficiency virus (HIV) infection. *Annals of Internal Medicine* **110**:727–733.

McKinney's Consolidated Laws of New York Annotated (1997) *HIV related testing*. Public Health Law Article 27-F, sec. 2781.

Peterson LM (1989) AIDS: the ethical dilemma for surgeons. *Law Medicine and Health Care* **17**:139–144.

Pomeroy C, Sandry J and Moldow DG (1994) HIV antibody testing: the gap between policy and practice. *Journal of Acquired Immune Deficiency Syndromes* **7**:816–822.

Quinn TC (1992) Screening for HIV infection—benefits and costs. *New England Journal of Medicine* **327**:486–488.

Sherer R (1988) Physician use of the HIV antibody test. *Journal of the American Medical Association* **259**:264–265.

Simonds RJ, Edlin BR and Rogers MF (1996) Preventing perinatal HIV transmission. *Journal of the American Medical Association* **276**:779–780.

Sontag D (1997) H. I. V. testing for newborns debated anew. *New York Times*, February 10 A1.

Swartz MS (1988) AIDS testing and informed consent. *Journal of Health Politics, Policy and Law* **13**:607–621.

Weiss R and Thier SO (1988) HIV testing is the answer—what's the question? *New England Journal of Medicine* **319**:1010–1012.

Wilkerson I (1989) Illinois legislature repeals requirement for prenuptial AIDS tests. *New York Times*, June 25: A12.

3

Should We Offer Predictive Tests for Fatal Inherited Diseases and, If So, How?

Susan M Wolf, Thomas G Horejsi

ABSTRACT

As the genetic basis for an increasing number of neurological disorders is identified, neurologists face the challenge of deciding what to tell their patients about genetics, when to offer genetic testing, and when to refer patients to genetic counsellors and specialists. These questions are particularly important in the case of fatal disorders. This essay examines the experience with Huntington's, Tay–Sachs, and Alzheimer's disease to offer recommendations.

INTRODUCTION

The age of neurogenetics is upon us. Genetic mutations have been identified for a variety of neurological disorders. As a result, neurologists now face questions of what to tell patients about the genetic underpinnings of their disease, when to offer genetic testing, and when to refer patients for genetic testing and counselling by others (Statement, 1996).

Neurologists are not alone in facing these challenges. The growing capacity to test adults, adolescents, children, fetuses, and even embryos for harmful mutations presents comparable challenges for all physicians. Yet neurological diseases have occupied a particularly important place in the debates over genetic testing. Chromosomal analysis for trisomy 21 has been available for decades and gene product analysis for Tay–Sachs disease (TSD) since the 1970s (Kaback *et al.*, 1993; Bird and Bennett, 1995; Jorde *et al.*, 1995, p. 108). Huntington's disease (HD), however, was one of the earliest disorders mapped to a particular chromosome using a DNA marker (Jorde *et al.*, 1995, p. 68). That 1983 feat facilitated genetic testing for HD, first through linkage analysis of families and then through molecular mutation analysis after the responsible mutation was identified in 1993. Today there is a large literature on HD testing, setting forth standards that have subsequently been widely applied to genetic testing for other disorders. TSD gene product and mutation analysis have also become widely accepted and an important model not only for individual genetic testing, but also for population screening. Lastly, Alzheimer's disease (AD) represents a genetic frontier, with identification of mutations associated with some forms of familial AD beginning in the 1990s and an active debate over whether genetic testing should be used for prediction and diagnosis. Though there are other neurological disorders whose genetic bases are known or becoming clear (see, e.g. Bird and Bennett, 1995; Rosenberg and Iannaccone, 1995), these three have provoked the most significant debates over genetic testing and screening. All three are marked by serious deterioration and ultimately death, so that our ability to predict the disorder may have a profound effect on patient and family decision making. HD is a late-onset disorder inherited dominantly. Much of the debate has focused on whether patients suffer harm from predictive testing, whether children and adolescents should undergo testing, and whether fetus and embryo testing is warranted, given that a newborn positive for HD can still expect several decades of good health. TSD is a recessively inherited disorder marked by devastating symptoms from infancy and death in childhood. Debate has centred on assuring voluntary testing and an ethical approach to population carrier screening. AD, another late-onset disorder like HD, has far more complex genetics, as discussed below. Multiple genes are involved, and testing asymptomatic individuals for APOE (the most prevalent of those genes) will at best reveal susceptibility to future disease rather than providing predictive certainty. Debate is under way concerning what diagnostic and predictive information APOE testing actually yields, how testing should consequently be used, and whether it should remain experimental or be used clinically.

This essay considers genetic testing for HD, TSD, and AD in order to illuminate the range of issues involved in deciding whether and when to test for fatal neurological disorders. We argue that genetic testing for each disease is appropriate under certain conditions. However, we further argue that serious problems currently plague genetic testing. These include the lack of a national mechanism for deciding when a test is ready for clinical use, insufficient physician knowledge about genetics, the lack of safeguards to assure the privacy of genetic information and protection against discrimination, and public misconceptions of the meaning of genetic information. In addition, the rise of multiplex testing for a wide array of conditions at once, and the direct marketing of genetic tests to patients are posing new and difficult challenges. All of these problems heighten the need for physician education and consideration of what constitutes appropriate use of these tests.

GENERAL PRINCIPLES GOVERNING GENETIC TESTING

The earliest literature offering ethical analysis of genetic tests focused on the population screening for phenylketonuria (PKU), sickle-cell disease, and TSD that began in the early 1960s (Committee, 1975; President's Commission, 1983, pp. 12, 31–5; Andrews *et al.*, 1994, pp. 39–44). Screening was accomplished by testing for gene products associated with the disease or carrier state. As noted above, in 1983 the HD mutation was mapped to a particular chromosome using a DNA marker. Subsequent genetic testing for HD (and, later, AD), before the precise mutation was identified, consisted of pedigree and linkage analysis. These required tracing the disease through generations in affected families, and searching for genetic markers known to be associated with the responsible mutation.

Early gene product screening and then linkage analysis produced a substantial body of literature (see, e.g. President's Commission, 1983; Huggins *et al.*, 1990). That literature distinguished between testing individuals at risk for or manifesting the disease, testing carriers in the case of recessively inherited disease, preconception testing of couples, and prenatal testing. Typically the literature recommended that testing be preceded by careful genetic counselling, detailed explanation of the test and what a positive or negative result would mean, protection of each individual's privacy even in the context of family genetic analysis, and assuring that each individual agreed to testing voluntarily. After testing, further counselling was recommended for both those testing positive and negative, and the privacy of the genetic information was to be protected.

With the identification of the mutations associated with HD, TSD, and AD, a new era of direct mutation analysis began, though such analysis may be used in conjunction with gene product testing or linkage analysis, depending on the disease at issue. Mutation analysis is generally less dependent on testing family members, though family testing may make mutation analysis more informative in some cases. Mutation analysis may also yield more definitive results.

Guidelines for current genetic testing and screening for HD, TSD, and AD have built on the earlier recommendations (see, e.g. Kaback *et al.*, 1993; McKinnon *et al.*, 1997; Post *et al.*, 1997). To be ethical, testing first requires a reliable test with adequate sensitivity, specificity, and positive predictive value, generating a low number of false positives. How much useful information the test yields will be in part a function of how penetrant the gene is in the population (what proportion of those with a positive genotype express the disease) and how variable the gene's expression is (the range in phenotypic manifestations of the mutation). For example, if a mutation is extremely variable in its expression, a positive test will yield less information about future disease than if the expression is more uniform.

The guidelines on molecular genetic testing continue to emphasize the importance of pre- and post-test genetic counselling, informed consent, voluntary choice, and protection of the privacy of the genetic information (see, e.g. Geller *et al.*, 1997). In the United States, when testing is done in the context of research, further precautions apply. An Institutional Review Board (IRB) or the equivalent must review the ethics of the proposed protocol (IRB review being required for all research that is federally funded, conducted in an institution assuring the federal government that all its research will be IRB-reviewed, or performed on drugs or devices requiring approval from the Food and Drug Administration (FDA)). Special requirements also apply to the consent forms used in research and the informed consent process.

There is a growing recognition that the law must adequately protect privacy and guard against discrimination (Wolf, 1995; Kapp, 1996; Yesley, 1997). In the United States, the law does not yet do this. Some safeguards are provided by state statutes on genetic testing (as in California, Minnesota, and Ohio, for example), the federal Americans with Disabilities Act (ADA), and a recent amendment to the Employees' Retirement Income Security Act (ERISA). However, it is widely agreed that these protections are inadequate, and numerous proposals have been made to improve safeguards (Yesley, 1997). For now, the possibility that others may gain access to a patient's private genetic information and use that information to discriminate must be discussed with the patient in the informed consent process. Explaining legal risks and safeguards accurately to patients is not a traditional role for physicians; advice from legal counsel and the development of brochures or other support material may be required.

Specific guidelines have emerged for testing minors, prenatal testing, and preimplantation diagnosis to test embryos before transferring them to the uterus in in-vitro fertilization (IVF) (see, e.g. Council, 1994; Ethics Committee, 1994; Wertz *et al.*, 1994). Testing minors has been generally disfavoured, on the basis that minors should have an opportunity to achieve majority and make their own considered decision about whether to undergo testing as an exercise of their autonomy. The literature recognizes exceptions and allows testing when it would have direct health benefit to the minor, as in the case of testing for familial adenomatous polyposis (FAP), which may warrant early removal of the colon to avert cancer (see, e.g. Wertz *et al.*, 1994). While one might argue that testing minors allows parents to offer their child reproductive counselling and general preparation for life, it is not clear that this benefit outweighs the associated harm (as direct health benefits may). Moreover, the argument seems too broad, as it would justify practically all genetic testing in minors. Still, in the absence of conclusive data on benefits and harm to minors, debate persists (Cohen, 1998).

Prenatal testing has provoked a large amount of literature, particularly as amniocentesis for women over 34 years of age at delivery has become routine (see, e.g. D'Alton and DeCherney, 1993; Council, 1994). Newer additional techniques include chorionic villus sampling, percutaneous umbilical blood sampling, and maternal serum testing. Discussion has focused on which patients should be offered prenatal testing, for what diseases and disorders, and with what counselling. Unlike genetic testing in non-pregnant adults and children, which requires only venipuncture, most prenatal testing is significantly invasive (maternal serum testing being the exception). Determination of which patients should be offered testing is affected by the risk of miscarriage or other harm to the woman or fetus, balanced against the informativeness of the test and severity of the disease or disorder. Thus the institutionalization of routine amniocentesis for women over 34 reflects the statistical fact that at 35 the risk of a genetic anomaly in the fetus begins to exceed the risk of miscarriage from the procedure, so that testing can confer net benefit.

Deciding what diseases or disorders to test for is controversial. Testing for conditions that will seriously affect the child, such as TSD and Down's syndrome, is widely accepted. But testing for late-onset disorders such as HD that in most cases will not affect the child until well into adulthood has prompted more dispute (Post, 1992; Lancaster *et al.*, 1996). Testing for conditions that are not diseases, such as sex (when not using sex to screen out X-linked disorders such as fragile X syndrome) is widely rejected (Council, 1994). While one could argue that parents-to-be should be able to test for anything they wish, health professionals object that in no other sphere do they simply do whatever the patient wants; professional judgements as to the appropriateness of offering a test are warranted. This controversy is fuelled in part by differences over the morality of abortion, a likely response by parents-to-be if a test reveals a trait unacceptable to them. But it is fuelled as well by differences over the role of non-medical concerns (such as fear that sex selection will encourage societal sexism) in professional medical judgements. Determining what counselling is appropriate is also bound up in the abortion debate to some extent. Though the literature on genetic counselling has favoured non-directiveness and acceptance of client values, there is growing debate over whether genetic counselling practice actually conforms to this ideal and whether the ideal itself should be re-examined (Caplan, 1993; Bartels *et al.*, 1997). Some argue that the question of whether a child should be born with devastating disease is not a matter on which counsellors should remain neutral, while others continue to advocate counsellor neutrality, since some parents-to-be will refuse abortion and value their child no matter what his or her condition.

Preimplantation genetic diagnosis of embryos is the newest of these genetic testing modalities (Ethics Committee, 1994; Pergament and Bonnicksen, 1994; Harper, 1996). Embryo biopsy (in which one or two cells are removed and analysed, usually at the 6–10-cell stage) has been used to test for disorders including cystic fibrosis and TSD, with normal children resulting (Handyside *et al.*, 1992; Gibbons *et al.*, 1995). Polar body biopsy is another technique; it removes less material and is less likely to interrupt the development of the embryo (Verlinsky *et al.*, 1990). These techniques require laboratory access to the embryo, so their application is limited to patients using IVF or willing to use IVF to perform embryo biopsy. Embryo biopsy is similar to prenatal testing in that net benefit is likely to accrue only when the informativeness of the test and the seriousness of the disease or disorder together justify the risk of the test interfering with the pregnancy or harming the child-to-be. This leads to similar discussion of what diseases or disorders should be tested for. Yet embryo biopsy differs from prenatal testing in that multiple embryos are being tested before transfer to the uterus and implantation, and indeed before individuation (given that embryos can still twin later) and development. Some have suggested that the moral status of the early embryo is less problematic than that of the fetus, and that failure to transfer is thus less problematic than abortion (Robertson, 1992; Ethics Committee, 1994). This provides more latitude for embryo testing. As yet, the technique of embryo testing has not been used as a broad screen, but rather to target a disorder of concern, such as cystic fibrosis. The potential for its future use to test for a wide range of disorders, however, will expand the debate.

Debate over the appropriateness of genetic testing in individuals overlaps with debate over genetic screening in populations. Though newborn screening for inborn metabolic disorders began in the early 1960s in the United States, it was not until the early 1970s that carrier screening began, focusing first on sickle-cell screening of African Americans (Reilly, 1975; President's Commission, 1983, pp. 12–23; Markel, 1992). The sickle-cell effort was very poorly designed, targeting a population already vulnerable to discrimination, and subjecting them to sometimes mandatory screening with inadequate counselling and grossly inadequate protection from further discrimination based on test results. The consequence was stigmatization, loss of employment, military exclusion, and other harm, often based on an individual being merely a carrier. This early sickle-cell screening remains a model of how not to perform screening.

Subsequent screening efforts, including those for TSD carrier status, have been marked by an insistence that the test be administered only to those voluntarily consenting and be accompanied by counselling (Kaback *et al.,* 1993). The best screening programmes have involved the population at risk in the planning process and have demonstrated cultural sensitivity. They have also paid careful attention to questions of patient privacy and confidentiality.

Progress in addressing ethical concerns in genetic testing and screening has grown out of an empirical literature reporting the experience of different programmes and researching specific questions, such as the psychological impact of HD testing. It has also grown out of a normative literature recommending guidelines to govern testing and screening. Some of these guidelines have issued from individuals, some from consensus groups and other projects, and some from professional societies. Yet there remains substantial concern that there is no national mechanism in the United States to decide when a test is ready for clinical application. Collins has argued that testing is not benign, but presents harm as well as benefits (Nowak, 1994). Yet testing remains largely unregulated (with the FDA exercising only limited jurisdiction and the Clinical Laboratory Improvement Act and Amendments (CLIA) governing only the rudiments of laboratory quality) (Andrews *et al.,* 1994, pp. 124–133; Holtzman *et al.,* 1997; Task Force, 1997). There has been significant recent controversy, for instance, over whether both cystic fibrosis and AD testing should expand into broader clinical application (see, e.g. Genetic Testing, 1997; Post *et al.,* 1997). Some authors have called for the creation of a national body to address such questions (Wilfond and Nolan, 1993; Andrews *et al.*, 1994, pp. 290–294; Holtzman *et al.*, 1997; Task Force, 1997). For now, the lack of an organized national process for determining when a test is ready for clinical use and in what populations places a heavy burden on individual physicians to decide when to offer testing.

TESTING FOR HUNTINGTON'S DISEASE

Genetic testing for HD has provoked a large amount of literature, with numerous guidelines and position papers (see, e.g. Guidelines, 1994; Hersch *et al.*, 1994; Bird and Bennett, 1995). Indeed, work on HD testing has often served as the model for other kinds of genetic testing (Tibben *et al.*, 1997a). Specific concerns remain: whether adult patients suffer psychological harm from predictive HD testing, whether children and adolescents should undergo testing, and whether prenatal testing of embryo and fetus is warranted.

The psychological impact of predictive HD testing flows from the severity of this late-onset disease. HD, which was first described by George Huntington in 1872, usually presents during the fourth or fifth decade of life. The disease is progressive, characterized by behavioural disturbance and chorea, and ends in death approximately 15 years from the time of onset (Bird, 1998). There is no known cure and treatment is extremely limited.

HD is an autosomal dominant disorder, so that if one parent is positive for the HD mutation, each child has a 50% chance of inheriting the mutation and thus manifesting the disorder. In 1993 the responsible mutation, an expansion of CAG repeats, was located on chromosome 4p16.3, so that direct mutation analysis is now available (Huntington's Disease Collaborative, 1993). The frequency of HD within the general population is listed as 1–10 in 10 000 across a large number of ethnic groups (Kremer *et al.*, 1994; Haque *et al.*, 1997).

The sensitivity of HD mutation analysis is now near 100%, and specificity at 100%, as a true positive result rests simply on the identification of CAG repeats (Kremer *et al.*, 1994). However, testing cannot tell a patient precisely when symptoms will arise. A higher number of CAG repeats seems to correlate with earlier age of onset (*Id.*). The number of CAG repeats can expand from one generation to the next within a family, in a pattern known as 'anticipation' (Kremer *et al.*, 1994; Jorde *et al.*, 1995, pp. 68, 76). A significant issue for genetic counsellors has been assessing risk in families that show intermediate range repeats (Alford *et al.*, 1996). Sporadic cases of HD have shown up in descendants of males who express a normal phenotype and possess an intermediate number of CAG repeats; expansion may render their offspring vulnerable (Ibid.).

A minority of at-risk adults seek testing (Lennox *et al.*, 1994; Kremer *et al.*, 1994; Bundey, 1997), and a quarter of those withdraw during pre-test counselling (Kremer *et al.*, 1994). A number of researchers have studied the psychological effects of testing (see, e.g. Wiggins *et al.*, 1992; Holloway *et al.*,

1994; Lawson *et al.*, 1996; Codori *et al.*, 1997; Tibben *et al.*, 1997b). When genetic testing for HD began, there was fear that testing would cause psychological harm. Indeed, some predicted that unfavourable results would lead to severe emotional reactions or suicide (Kessler *et al.*, 1987). Numerous follow-up studies suggest that the net effect of testing is generally positive, and that eliminating uncertainty may yield psychological benefit (see, e.g. Wiggins *et al.*, 1992; Bundey, 1997; Codori *et al.*, 1997; Tibben *et al.*, 1997b). However, test results can cause short-term psychological distress, which seems to moderate over time (Codori *et al.*, 1997; Tibben *et al.*, 1997b). Significant adverse effects have been reported in some cases, but with a low overall rate of psychiatric reactions (Wiggins *et al.*, 1992; Decruyenaere *et al.*, 1996; Codori *et al.*, 1997; Tibben *et al.*, 1997b). Thus, physician concern that patients generally are not able to tolerate HD testing seems unwarranted, even though problematic cases may arise. Genetic counselling is essential and further psychological counselling should be available. Patients should also be counselled about potential problems in maintaining the privacy of their test results and avoiding discrimination, especially in employment and insurance.

Testing children and adolescents for HD raises more acute concerns. Most authorities discourage it (Bloch and Hayden, 1990; Harper and Clarke, 1990; Guidelines, 1994; Report, 1994; American Society, 1995). While the illness or genetic testing of a relative may raise the question of the minor's status, and parents may wish to counsel the minor about future reproduction, the child or adolescent will usually derive no immediate health benefit from the knowledge. Instead, the minor may suffer psychological harm from the burden of receiving a positive test result, from 'survivor guilt' associated with receiving a negative result, and from being deprived of the opportunity to make an autonomous decision upon achieving the age of majority. Even a minor who shows neurological and behavioural changes suspected to be rare childhood-onset HD can be diagnosed without genetic testing (Bloch and Hayden, 1990; Report, 1994). There are, however, few data on the impact of HD testing on minors (Michie and Marteau, 1996). Beyond concerns over psychological harm, the child may become uninsurable and suffer other forms of life-long discrimination as a result of testing. Testing has been endorsed by some commentators in exceptional circumstances, such as when an adolescent is reproductively active or demonstrates a compelling wish to know even after counselling (Wertz *et al.*, 1994; American Society, 1995; Binedell *et al.*, 1996).

Testing is widely accepted for adults making reproductive choices (Council, 1994). Thus, at-risk couples may seek testing for themselves when planning a pregnancy. Testing in fetuses and embryos is more controversial, since even individuals with the mutation can expect several decades of healthy life (Post, 1992; Post *et al.*, 1992; Schulman *et al.*, 1996). However, because HD is a devastating and ultimately fatal disorder that cuts life expectancy in half, there are strong reasons to make testing available to couples and to defer to their judgement on whether to use it. Both law and ethics have recognized the powerful claims of pregnant women and reproducing couples to reproductive liberty. Genetic testing, especially amniocentesis, has already become a common part of the reproductive process. Interfering with access to genetic testing and decisions based on that testing thus requires an extremely strong justification.

TESTING AND SCREENING FOR TAY–SACHS DISEASE

TSD differs from HD in several critical ways. Because it is recessively inherited, individuals may be carriers and not know it. Thus, great effort has been devoted to identifying carriers through reproductive testing and population screening. Second, TSD is most common among Jews of Ashkenazi descent (Triggs-Raine et al., 1990). TSD has a carrier rate of 1/31 among Jews, compared to 1/277 among non-Jewish individuals (Kaback et al., 1993), though a genetic isolate of French Canadians in Eastern Quebec also has a high frequency (Andermann et al., 1977; Hechtman and Kaplan, 1993). Thus, screening has been concentrated among populations with a relatively high carrier frequency. Third, the most common form of TSD shows no delay in onset, with symptoms beginning in early childhood and death usually resulting by 3–5 years of age. The severity and early onset of the disease have contributed to the wide acceptance of adult carrier screening, as well as prenatal and preimplantation testing to detect homozygous (and therefore affected) fetuses and embryos.

Over a century ago, Warren Tay and Bernard Sachs described a disorder characterized by cerebral degeneration, blindness, and loss of motor function (Hechtman and Kaplan, 1993). By 1969 it was known that TSD is characterized by a deficiency in the activity of the lysosomal hydrolase β-hexosaminidase A (HEX A), resulting in the accumulation of G_{M2} ganglioside within neuronal lysosomes (Kaback et al., 1993). In addition to the classically defined infantile TSD, there also exist juvenile- and adult-onset G_{M2} gangliosidoses (Kaback et al., 1993). There are no effective treatments for TSD.

Genetic testing has revealed a range of mutations associated with TSD. Among patients with classic infantile-onset TSD, nearly 40 different mutations have been identified across a number of ethnic origins (Hechtman and Kaplan, 1993; Kaback et al., 1993). However, in the Ashkenazi Jewish population of North America, three mutations (two correlated with infantile TSD and one with adult) account for 92–98% of the mutant alleles (Kaback et al., 1993).

Given the number of mutations involved, widespread testing is most feasible by analysis of the gene product, supplemented by direct mutation analysis in the case of a positive gene product result. Gene product analysis is less costly and should identify the vast majority of all individuals with mutations with few false negatives, though special procedures are required for accurate testing in pregnant women (Triggs-Raine et al., 1990; Hechtman and Kaplan, 1993; Kaback et al., 1993). Follow-up mutation analysis has been recommended for all individuals testing positive for the gene product, in part to rule out pseudodeficient mutations (Kaback *et al.*, 1993). TSD carriers can be identified through gene product analysis, mutation analysis, or both with 99% detectability (Eng *et al.*, 1997).

Prenatal screening and carrier screening programmes have been initiated throughout the North American Ashkenazi Jewish population. These have resulted in a significant decrease in TSD rates since 1970 (Kaback *et al.*, 1993). TSD screening has avoided many of the pitfalls that deeply marred early sickle-cell screening (Kaback *et al.*, 1993). Although both screening efforts targeted populations historically vulnerable to prejudice and discrimination, TSD screening has been strictly voluntary. There has also been a concerted effort to offer adequate counselling and education. The contrast between the sickle-cell and TSD experience highlights the critical role that voluntary consent, genetic counselling, and community education play. In addition, TSD programmes have often involved rabbis and community leaders in the planning process, contributing further to acceptance and success.

TESTING FOR ALZHEIMER'S DISEASE

Alzheimer's disease (AD) is another late-onset disease like HD, but with far more complex genetics. AD was first described in 1907 by Alois Alzheimer. It affects about 25% of all persons over the age of 85 (some offer an even higher percentage), is the prevalent cause of dementia in the elderly, and is the fourth leading cause of death in the US (Evans *et al.*, 1989; Post *et al.*, 1997; Rosenberg, 1997; Bird, 1998). AD is characterized by memory loss followed by slowly progressing dementia, often culminating in a profound loss of cognitive abilities, becoming bedridden, and death. The usual course of AD is 8–10 years but may be between 1 and 25 years (Bird, 1998). There is no specific treatment for AD, though at least one drug seems to slow disease progression in some patients (Farlow, 1997). Most therapeutic efforts have been devoted to managing the long-term behavioural and neurological problems.

AD presents a more complicated genetic picture than HD or TSD, and its genetics are not yet fully understood. AD is a disorder that may result from mutations at several loci and in which environmental factors may play a role. Four genes have been implicated thus far: PS1 (presenilin-1), PS2 (presenilin-2), APP (amyloid precursor protein), and APOE (apolipoprotein) (Rosenberg, 1997). The first three yield autosomal dominant mutations causally associated with early-onset AD (in the 40s or 50s), which constitutes 1–5% of all AD cases. Even in these autosomal dominant cases, environment and other genetic factors may affect age of onset (Frisoni and Trabucchi, 1997). Testing for these mutations raises issues similar to those in HD, though they are made more complex by the possibility of variable expression of AD in individual patients (Post *et al.*, 1997).

APOE, on the other hand, is a susceptibility gene that increases the likelihood of developing AD, but does not predict it to a certainty. Researchers found an association between AD and the APOE ε4 allele in 1993 (Strittmatter *et al.*, 1993). The allele is thought to be associated with 10–40% of all AD (Frisoni and Trabucchi, 1997). The APOE ε4 allele has a frequency of about 15% in populations of European ancestry (National Institute, 1996; Relkin *et al.*, 1996). The ε4 allele is associated both with higher risk of AD and earlier onset. Lifetime risk of AD has been estimated at 9% with no ε4 allele and 29% with at least one (Seshadri *et al.*, 1995; Post *et al.*, 1997). Some estimates are higher (Corder *et al.*, 1993). Having one or two copies of the APOE mutation thus increases risk, but it does not tell the individual patient whether disease will develop or when (Post *et al.*, 1997). Persons with no copies of the ε4 mutation can develop AD, while homozygotes for the mutation may never develop the disorder (Post *et al.*, 1997). APOE allele frequencies have been established in a variety of populations (Relkin *et al.*, 1996). Commercial testing for APOE became available in 1994 (Post *et al.*, 1997). Some patients have been tested in the context of cardiovascular, not AD, assessment, raising difficult questions of what they should be told about their risk for AD (National Institute, 1996; Wachbroit, 1998).

Interpreting APOE testing, assessing risk of AD, and predicting severity and onset are thus complex. Family history remains one of the most telling factors in risk assessment (National Institute, 1996). Further research should elucidate how age, sex, ethnicity, other genetic factors, and environmental exposures may modify risk (National Institute, 1996; Relkin *et al.*, 1996).

Appropriate use of APOE testing remains controversial. Several position papers and guidelines have been published (see, e.g. American College, 1995; Medical and Scientific Advisory Committee, 1995; Relkin *et al.*, 1996; McKinnon *et al.*, 1997; Post *et al.*, 1997). APOE testing to diagnose AD has generally been disapproved, though some recent articles suggest that data may eventually support this use (American College, 1995; Lovestone, 1996; Post *et al.*, 1997). It is as yet unclear whether the APOE/AD association is strong enough in various ethnic groups to make a positive APOE test yield significant diagnostic information (Breitner, 1996; Post *et al.*, 1997). Studies suggest that the APOE test lacks the sensitivity and specificity necessary to be used alone for diagnosis (American College, 1995; see also Relkin *et al.*, 1996). Moreover, clinicians can use a variety of tests and criteria to exclude other causes of dementia and diagnose AD without genetic testing (Post *et al.*, 1997). There is also discussion of whether APOE testing can identify patients more likely to respond to certain therapies (American College, 1995; Frisoni and Trabucchi, 1997).

APOE testing to predict future risk of AD in asymptomatic individuals is currently not recommended, as a positive test has limited utility in predicting disease (Breitner, 1996; National Institute, 1996; Relkin *et al.*, 1996; Post *et al.*, 1997). Current genetic tests lack the sensitivity and specificity to be adequately informative (American College, 1995). Moreover, because AD is a late-onset and severe disorder, there is substantial concern over the psychological impact of predictive testing (Post, 1994; Tibben *et al.*, 1997a). Indeed, the psychological concerns are greater in the case of AD than HD, since adverse consequences are more likely to result from an uninformative test, inaccurate interpretation of results, and inadequate genetic counselling (Relkin *et al.*, 1996). Because the genetics of AD are complex, the potential for misunderstanding is great. The lack of established predictive usefulness, very late onset of AD, and potential for misunderstanding should militate against APOE testing in minors, fetuses, and embryos at present.

Despite recommendations against testing asymptomatic individuals in the general population, APOE testing has been conducted in both clinical and research settings (Post *et al.*, 1997). Some commentators have argued that predictive testing should only be used in research contexts at present (American College, 1995; Tibben *et al.*, 1997a). This issue demonstrates the lack of a centralized national mechanism for determining when a genetic test is ready to be used outside research. The literature debating the wisdom of cystic fibrosis carrier screening in the general population similarly bemoans the absence of such a mechanism (Wilfond and Nolan, 1993). It means that testing may well be instituted before the benefits justify such use, as seems to be happening with APOE testing to predict disease.

RECOMMENDATIONS AND REMAINING PROBLEMS

Analysis of genetic testing for HD, TSD, and AD yields several recommendations for genetic testing for fatal neurological disorders. First, testing is appropriate under certain circumstances. That means that neurologists and other clinicians must know enough about the genetics of these disorders and about the prevalent recommendations for testing to know when to offer testing, when to refer patients for testing and counselling, and how to respond to patients' queries about the genetics.

Yet data suggest that many physicians lack adequate genetic knowledge (Hofman *et al.*, 1993; Seshadri *et al.*, 1995; Giardiello *et al.*, 1997; Stephenson, 1997). One study found that almost one-third of physicians interpreting test results for mutations relating to familial adenomatous polyposis (FAP) misinterpreted the results (Giardiello *et al.*, 1997). The challenge of genetic literacy will not be met simply by increasing referrals to genetic counsellors and specialists. Cost and other barriers may impede access and, in any case, there will soon be too few counsellors and medical geneticists to meet the demand for testing and services (Collins, 1997). Data also indicate that primary care physicians are divided between those who refer patients to genetic counsellors and those who perform counselling themselves, even though physicians who do it themselves are more directive than genetic counsellors (Geller *et al.*, 1993). This suggests that physicians may require training not only in genetics but also in the provision of genetic services. It seems clear that medical schools and continuing medical education will have to offer more genetics education (Andrews *et al.*, 1994, pp. 216–223). Current computer technology can assist, at least in conveying genetics information, through resources such as CD ROM programs and Internet sites (Sikorski and Peters, 1997; Stephenson, 1997).

A second recommendation is that clinicians must be cautious in offering and urging that patients take a genetic test. As Collins has suggested, testing is not simply the benign acquisition of knowledge (Nowak, 1994). It can have serious psychological and social effects and alter the course of a patient's life. Patients may request testing with only a dim understanding of what test results would mean. Indeed, scholars have written about a widespread tendency toward genetic reductionism, that is, assuming simplistically that all sorts of traits— from vulnerability to cancer to IQ—are genetically determined (Lippman, 1991; Dreyfuss and Nelkin, 1992; Rose, 1995; Wolf, 1995). Misunderstanding of genetics is rampant. This virtually guarantees that clinicians will receive requests for inappropriate genetic testing and will see patients who misconstrue their test results, sometimes despite genetic counselling. Clinicians must educate themselves to dispel such misunderstanding.

This will be particularly important in the face of commercial efforts to promote genetic tests directly to patients. A federal task force has recently discouraged direct advertising of predictive genetic tests because of concern that informational material may be inaccurate and cause harm (Task Force, 1997). Others, including a British advisory committee, have been more receptive (Advisory Committee, 1997; Editorial, 1997). In any case, direct advertising may mean that patients demand genetic tests from their physicians without complete and accurate information. Physicians must be prepared to discuss testing options accurately with their patients and dispel misconceptions. A further related concern is that some laboratories may run genetic tests at the patient's request with no involvement of the treating physician (Task Force, 1997). While some commentators decry the potential here for misinformed decisions and harm to the patient, others champion a right to know (Editorial, 1997; Task Force, 1997). As debate continues, physicians should make an effort to uncover and address their patients' genetic concerns in order to offer patients the benefit of their expertise.

Even when direct advertising and marketing are not in the picture, inappropriate testing can certainly occur. Reducing inappropriate testing requires physicians and their institutions to participate in an orderly process of introducing new tests. The laboratory identification of a mutation associated with a disorder does not make a test ready for clinical introduction (Wilfond and Nolan, 1993; Holtzman *et al.*, 1997; Task Force, 1997). Assessment of a test's sensitivity, specificity, and predictive value is part of the research process that should precede clinical application. In the research phase an IRB or comparable body should review the ethics of the proposed research protocol, research subjects should go through a more elaborate and protective consent process than in routine clinical practice, and the study's results should be published for public scrutiny and debate.

A third recommendation is that such research should feed into a national process for assessing new genetic tests and determining when they are ready for clinical use. Currently the process is largely unregulated in the United States. Some laboratory standards exist under the Clinical Laboratory Improvement Act and Amendments (CLIA), while the FDA exerts control over genetic test kits but not services; that leaves a substantial gap (Andrews *et al.*, 1994, pp. 124–133; Holtzman *et al.*, 1997; Task Force, 1997). As noted above, for example, there has been extensive debate over whether to begin offering cystic fibrosis carrier screening beyond families affected by the illness, and an NIH consensus panel recently began advocating such testing under certain circumstances (Genetic Testing, 1997). But there is no formal national process for making this kind of determination, whether it be through a governmental advisory committee, regulatory body, or some other mechanism (Wilfond and Nolan, 1993; Andrews *et al.*, 1994, pp. 290–294; Holtzman *et al.*, 1997; Task Force, 1997). The debate over testing for AD could certainly benefit from such a process.

A fourth recommendation is that once a test is suitable for clinical use, testing must be voluntary after an informed consent process and genetic counselling. Though this set of requirements is familiar, clinical fulfillment remains a challenge. Formal genetic counselling and written informed consent may simply be omitted, especially when the patient is already symptomatic (Giardiello *et al.*, 1997). Even if counselling occurs, the literature documents substantial difficulties in communicating genetic information, particularly as it is characterized by probabilities and uncertainties (see, e.g. Lippman-Hand and Fraser, 1979a–c; Lippman, 1991). Communicating information about a disease as genetically complex as AD magnifies the challenge.

One of the greatest challenges to fulfilling the requirement of voluntary testing after informed consent and counselling is the rise of multiplex testing. This can involve testing a patient simultaneously for a number of mutations relating to different conditions. Multiplex testing can also be used for population screening. However, it may be very difficult to explain all the mutations being tested for, to counsel the patient on the limitations of each test, and to obtain informed consent to the package. The problem is exacerbated by the fact that different mutations tested for may raise quite different issues: some mutations may cause disease while others merely confer susceptibility or indicate carrier status, some may be associated with current disease while others predict late-onset disorders, and so on. Communicating all of this information to the patient to obtain informed consent may be daunting. A number of recommendations have been made to address these problems, including grouping together only tests that raise similar issues, or eliciting generic consent before testing and providing detailed explanation later for only those mutations for which the patient tests positive, or simply insisting on informed consent to each test as a prerequisite to multiplex testing (Andrews *et al.*, 1994; Elias and Annas, 1994; Council, 1998).

An additional problem in obtaining informed consent for genetic testing is that the clinician must address the patient's vulnerability to invasions of privacy and to discrimination based on genetic information. This requires knowledge of what protections exist for the privacy of genetic information and what safeguards currently prevent discrimination. In fact, the current US protections and safeguards are inadequate, though state and federal efforts to remedy this are under way (Wolf, 1995; Kapp, 1996; Yesley, 1997). Yet many patients remain unaware of the risk of discrimination (Tibben *et al.*, 1997a), and presumably are also unaware of substantial gaps in the protection of the privacy of their genetic information. Materials informing patients of these problems are sorely needed, as are improvements in the legal safeguards.

These recommendations present an agenda not only for individual physicians in their practice, but for genetic counsellors and specialists in their patient care, for researchers introducing and improving genetic tests, for professional societies offering guidelines on genetic testing, for policy makers deciding what national mechanism should advise on genetic tests, and for law makers improving safeguards for patient privacy and protections against discrimination. Genetics has already become an unavoidable part of neurological practice, with the identification of mutations associated with HD, TSD, AD, and other disorders. With tremendous effort now going into mapping and sequencing the human genome, the role of genetics will only grow. Every neurologist will face the question of whether to test or recommend testing for fatal neurological disorders. Yet the potential harm resulting from genetic testing—including permanent stigmatization and uninsurability, as well as prediction of disease and disability not only for the patient but also for future generations—exceeds that following most other forms of clinical testing. Genetic knowledge, careful reflection, and advice from professional and national bodies are critical to meeting this challenge.

Acknowledgements

The authors thank Dianne Bartels, Ellen Clayton, Linda Emanuel, Jeffrey Kahn, Bonnie LeRoy, and Adam Zeman for helpful comments; Robert Cook-Deegan, Pete Magee, and Stephen Post for addressing queries; and Dana Shenker of the University of Minnesota Law School for able research assistance. The Center for Bioethics at the University of Minnesota provided generous support.

REFERENCES

Advisory Committee on Genetic Testing (1997) *Code of Practice and Guidance on Human Genetic Testing Services Supplied Direct to the Public*. London: Department of Health.

Alford RL, Ashizawa T, Jankovic J et al. (1996) Molecular detection of new mutations: resolution of ambiguous results and complex genetic counseling issues in Huntington disease. *American Journal of Medical Genetics* **66**:281–286.

American College of Medical Genetics/American Society of Human Genetics Working Group on ApoE and Alzheimer Disease (1995) Statement on use of apolipoprotein E testing for Alzheimer disease. *Journal of the American Medical Association* **274 (20)**:1627–1629.

American Society of Human Genetics Board of Directors and The American College of Medical Genetics Board of Directors (1995) ASHG/ACMG Report: points to consider: ethical, legal, and psychosocial implications of genetic testing in children and adolescents. *American Journal of Human Genetics* **57**:1233–1241.

Andermann E, Scriver CR, Wolfe LS *et al.* (1977) Genetic variants of Tay-Sachs disease: Tay-Sachs disease and Sandhoff's disease in French Canadians, juvenile Tay-Sachs disease in Lebanese Canadians, and a Tay-Sachs screening program in the French-Canadian population. *Progress in Clinical and Biological Research* **18**:161–188.

Andrews LB, Fullarton JE, Holtzman NA *et al.* (eds) (1994) *Assessing Genetic Risks: Implications for Health and Social Policy.* Washington, DC: National Academy Press.

Bartels DM, LeRoy BS, McCarthy P *et al.* (1997) Nondirectiveness in genetic counseling: a survey of practitioners. *American Journal of Medical Genetics* **72**:172–179.

Binedell J, Soldan JR, Scourfield J *et al.* (1996) Huntington's disease predictive testing: the case for an assessment approach to requests from adolescents. *Journal of Medical Genetics* **33**:912–918.

Bird TD (1998) Alzheimer's disease and other primary dementias. In: *Harrison's Principles of Internal Medicine* (ed. AS Fauci), Vol. 2, 14th edn, pp. 2348–2356. New York: McGraw-Hill.

Bird TD and Bennett RL (1995) Why do DNA testing? Practical and ethical implications of new neurogenetic tests. *Annals of Neurology* **38**:141–146.

Bloch M and Hayden MR (1990) Opinion: predictive testing for Huntington disease in childhood: challenges and implications. *American Journal of Human Genetics* **46**:1–4.

Breitner JSC (1996) APOE genotyping and Alzheimer's disease. *Lancet* **347**:1184–1185.

Bundey S (1997) Few psychological consequences of presymptomatic testing for Huntington disease. *Lancet* **349**:4.

Caplan AL (1993) Neutrality is not morality: the ethics of genetic counseling. In: *Prescribing Our Future: Ethical Challenges in Genetic Counseling* (eds DM Bartels, BS LeRoy, AL Caplan), pp. 149–165. New York: Aldine De Gruyter.

Codori AM, Slavney PR, Young C *et al.* (1997) Predictors of psychological adjustment to genetic testing for Huntington's disease. *Health Psychology* **16**:36–50.

Cohen CB (1998) Wrestling with the future: should we test children for adult-onset genetic conditions? *Kennedy Institute of Ethics Journal* **8**:111–130.

Collins FS (1997) Preparing health professionals for the genetic revolution. *Journal of the American Medical Association* **278**:1285–1286.

Committee for the Study of Inborn Errors of Metabolism, National Research Council (1975) *Genetic Screening: Programs, Principles, and Research.* Washington, DC: National Academy of Sciences.

Corder EH, Saunders AM, Strittmatter WJ *et al.* (1993) Gene dose of apolipoprotein E type 4 allele and the risk of Alzheimer's disease in late onset families. *Science* **261**:921–923.

Council on Ethical and Judicial Affairs, American Medical Association (1994) Ethical issues related to prenatal genetic testing. *Archives of Family Medicine* **3**:633–642.

Council on Ethical and Judicial Affairs, American Medical Association (1998) Multiplex genetic testing. *Hastings Center Report* **28 (4)**:15–21.

D'Alton ME and DeCherney AH (1993) Prenatal diagnosis. *New England Journal of Medicine* **328**:114–120.

Decruyenaere M, Evers-Kiebooms G, Boogaerts A *et al.* (1996) Prediction of psychological functioning one year after the predictive test for Huntington's disease and impact of the test result on reproductive decision making. *Journal of Medical Genetics* **33**:737–743.

Dreyfuss RC and Nelkin D (1992) The jurisprudence of genetics. *Vanderbilt Law Review* **45**:313–348.

Editorial (1997) Knowing your genes. *Lancet* **350**:969–970.

Elias S and Annas GJ (1994) Generic consent for genetic screening. *New England Journal of Medicine* **330**:1611–1613.

Eng C, Schechter C, Robinowitz J *et al.* (1997) Prenatal genetic carrier testing using triple disease screening. *Journal of the American Medical Association* **278**:1268–1272.

Ethics Committee, American Fertility Society (1994) Preimplantation genetic diagnosis. In: *Ethical considerations of assisted reproductive technologies. Fertility and Sterility* **62 (suppl. 1)**: 60S–3.

Evans DA, Funkenstein HH, Albert MS *et al.* (1989) Prevalence of Alzheimer's disease in a community of older persons: higher than previously reported. *Journal of the American Medical Association* **262**:2551–2556.

Farlow MR (1997) Alzheimer's disease: clinical implications of the apolipoprotein E genotype. *Neurology* **48 (suppl. 6)**:S30–4.

Frisoni GB and Trabucchi M (1997) Clinical rationale of genetic testing in dementia. *Journal of Neurology, Neurosurgery and Psychiatry* **62**:217–221.

Geller G, Tambor ES, Chase GA *et al.* (1993) Incorporation of genetics in primary care practice: will physicians do the counseling and will they be directive? *Archives of Family Medicine* 2:1119–1125.

Geller G, Botkin JR, Green MJ *et al.* (1997) Genetic testing for susceptibility to adult-onset cancer: the process and content of informed consent. *Journal of the American Medical Association* 227:1467–1474.

Genetic testing for cystic fibrosis (1997) *NIH Consensus Statement* April 14–16; **15 (4)**:1–37.

Giardiello FM, Brensinger JD, Petersen GM *et al.* (1997) The use and interpretation of commercial APC gene testing for familial adenomatous polyposis. *New England Journal of Medicine* 336: 823–827.

Gibbons WE, Gitlin SA, Lanzendorf SE *et al.* (1995) Preimplantation genetic diagnosis for Tay-Sachs disease: successful pregnancy after pre-embryo biopsy and gene amplification by polymerase chain reaction. *Fertility and Sterility* 63:723–728.

Guidelines for the molecular genetics predictive test in Huntington's disease (1994). *Neurology* 44:1533–1536.

Handyside AH, Lesko JG, Tarin JJ *et al.* (1992) Birth of a normal girl after in vitro fertilization and preimplantation diagnostic testing for cystic fibrosis. *New England Journal of Medicine* 327:905–909.

Haque NS, Borghesani P, Isacson O *et al.* (1997) Therapeutic strategies for Huntington's disease based on a molecular understanding of the disorder. *Molecular Medicine Today* 3 **(4)**:175–183.

Harper JC (1996) Preimplantation diagnosis of inherited disease by embryo biopsy: an update of world figures. *Journal of Assisted Reproduction* 13:90–95.

Harper PS and Clarke A (1990) Should we test children for 'adult' genetic diseases? *Lancet* 335:1205–1206.

Hechtman P and Kaplan F (1993) Tay-Sachs disease screening and diagnosis: evolving technologies. *DNA Cell Biology* 12:651–665.

Hersch S, Jones R, Koroshetz W *et al.* (1994) The neurogenetics genie: testing for the Huntington's disease mutation. *Neurology* 44:1369–1373.

Hofman KJ, Tambor ES, Chase GA *et al.* (1993) Physicians' knowledge of genetics and genetic tests. *Academic Medicine* 68:625–632.

Holloway S, Mennie M, Crosbie A *et al.* (1994) Predictive testing for Huntington disease: social characteristics and knowledge of applicants, attitudes to the test procedure and decisions made after testing. *Clinical Genetics* 46:175–180.

Holtzman NA, Murphy PD, Watson MS *et al.* (1997) Predictive genetic testing: from basic research to clinical practice. *Science* 278:602–605.

Huggins M, Bloch M, Kanani S *et al.* (1990) Ethical and legal dilemmas arising during predictive testing for adult-onset disease: the experience of Huntington disease. *American Journal of Human Gentics* 47:4–12.

Huntington's Disease Collaborative Research Group (1993) A novel gene containing a trinucleotide repeat that is expanded and unstable on Huntington's disease chromosomes. *Cell* 72:971–983.

Jorde LB, Carey JC and White RL (eds) (1995) *Medical Genetics.* St. Louis, MO: Mosby.

Kaback M, Lim-Steele J, Dabholkar D *et al.* (1993) Tay-Sachs disease—carrier screening, prenatal diagnosis, and the molecular era: an international perspective, 1970 to 1993. *Journal of the American Medical Association* 270:2307–2315.

Kapp M (1996) Medicolegal, employment, and insurance issues in APOE genotyping and Alzheimer's disease. *Annals of the New York Academy of Sciences* 802:139–148.

Kessler S, Field T, Worth L *et al.* (1987) Attitudes of persons at risk for Huntington disease toward predictive testing. *American Journal of Medical Genetics* 26:259–270.

Kremer B, Glodberg P, Andrew SE *et al.* (1994) A worldwide study of the Huntington's disease mutation, the sensitivity and specificity of measuring CAG repeats. *New England Journal of Medicine* 330(20):1401–1406.

Lancaster JM, Wiseman RW, Berchuck A (1996) An inevitable dilemma: prenatal testing for mutations in the BRCA1 breast-ovarian cancer susceptibility gene. *Obstetrics and Gynecology* 87: 306–309.

Lawson K, Wiggins S, Green T *et al.* (1996) Adverse psychological events occurring in the first year after predictive testing for Huntington's disease. *Journal of Medical Genetics* 33:856–862.

Lennox A, Karlinsky H, Meschino W *et al.* (1994) Molecular genetic predictive testing for Alzheimer's disease: deliberations and preliminary recommendations. *Alzheimer Disease and Associated Disorders* 8:126–147.

Lippman A (1991) Prenatal genetic testing and screening: constructing needs and reinforcing inequities. *American Journal of Law and Medicine* 17:15–50.

Lippman-Hand A and Fraser FC (1979a) Genetic counseling: provision and reception of information. *American Journal of Medical Genetics* 3:113–127.

Lippman-Hand A and Fraser FC (1979b) Genetic counseling—the postcounseling period: I. parents' perceptions of uncertainty. *American Journal of Medical Genetics* 4:51–71.

Lippman-Hand A and Fraser FC (1979c) Genetic counseling—the postcounseling period: II. making reproductive choices. *American Journal of Medical Genetics* 4:73–87.

Lovestone S (1996) The genetics of Alzheimer's disease—new opportunities and new challenges. *International Journal of Geriatric Psychiatry* 11:491–497.

Markel H (1992) The stigma of disease: implications of genetic screening. *American Journal of Medicine* 93:209–215.

McKinnon WC, Baty BJ, Bennett RL *et al.* (1997) Predisposition genetic testing for late-onset disorders in adults: a position paper of the National Society of Genetic Counselors. *Journal of the American Medical Association* 278:1217–1220.

Medical and Scientific Advisory Committee of Alzheimer's Disease International (1995) Consensus statement on predictive testing for Alzheimer's disease. *Alzheimer Disease and Associated Disorders* 9:182–187.

Michie S and Marteau TM (1996) Predictive genetic testing in children: the need for psychological research. *British Journal of Health Psychology* 1:3–14.

National Institute on Aging/Alzheimer's Association Working Group (1996) Apolipoprotein E genotyping in Alzheimer's disease. *Lancet* 347:1091–1095.

Nowak R (1994) Genetic testing set for takeoff. *Science* 265:464–467.

Pergament E and Bonnicksen A (1994) Preimplantation genetics: a case for prospective action. *American Journal of Medical Genetics* 52:151–157.

Post S (1992) Huntington's disease: prenatal screening for late onset disease. *Journal of Medical Ethics* 18:75–78.

Post S (1994) Genetics, ethics, and Alzheimer disease. *Journal of the American Genetics Society* 42:782–786.

Post SG, Botkin JR and Whitehouse P (1992) Selective abortion for familial Alzheimer disease? *Obstetrics and Gynecology* 79:794–798.

Post SG, Whitehouse PJ, Binstock RH *et al.* (1997) The clinical introduction of genetic testing for Alzheimer disease: an ethical perspective. *Journal of the American Medical Association* 277(10):832–836.

President's Commission for the Study of Ethical Problems in Medicine and Biomedical and Behavioral Research (1983) *Screening and Counseling for Genetic Conditions.* Washington, DC: US Government Printing Office.

Reilly P (1975) State supported mass genetic screening programs. In: *Genetics and the Law* (eds A Milunsky and GJ Annas), pp. 159–184. New York: Plenum.

Relkin NR, Kwon YJ, Tsai J *et al.* (1996) The National Institute on Aging/Alzheimer's Association recommendations on the application of apolipoprotein E genotyping to Alzheimer's disease. *Annals of the New York Academy of Sciences* 802:149–171.

Report of a Working Party of the Clinical Genetics Society (UK) (1994) The genetic testing of children. *Journal of Medical Genetics* 31:785–797.

Robertson JA (1992) Ethical and legal issues in preimplantation genetic screening. *Fertility and Sterility* 57:1–11.

Rose S (1995) The rise of neurogenic determinism. *Nature* 373:380–382.

Rosenberg R (1997) Molecular neurogenetics: the genome is settling the issue. *Journal of the American Medical Association* 278:1282–1284.

Rosenberg RN and Iannaccone ST (1995) The prevention of neurogenetic disease. *Archives of Neurology* 52:356–362.

Schulman JD, Black SH, Handyside A *et al.* (1996) Preimplantation genetic testing for Huntington disease and certain other dominantly inherited disorders. *Clinical Genetics* 49:57–58.

Seshadri S, Drachman DA and Lippa CF (1995) Apolipoprotein E ε4 allele and the lifetime risk of Alzheimer's disease: what physicians know, and what they should know. *Archives of Neurology* **52**:1074–1079.

Sikorski R and Peters R (1997) Genomic medicine: internet resources for medical genetics. *Journal of the American Medical Association* **278**:1212–1213.

Statement of the Practice Committee Genetics Testing Task Force of the American Academy of Neurology (1996) Practice parameter: genetic testing alert. *Neurology* **47**:1343–1344.

Stephenson J (1997) As discoveries unfold, a new urgency to bring genetic literacy to physicians. *Journal of the American Medical Association* **278**:1225–1226.

Strittmatter WJ, Saunders AM, Schmechel D *et al.* (1993) Apolipoprotein E: high-avidity binding to betaamyloid and increased frequency of type 4 allele in late-onset familial Alzheimer disease. *Proceedings of the National Academy of Sciences of the USA* **90**:1977–1981.

Task Force on Genetic Testing (1997) *Promoting Safe and Effective Genetic Testing in the United States, Final Report.* <http://www.nhgri.nih.gov/Elsi/TFGT_final/>

Tibben A, Stevens M, de Wert GMWR *et al.* (1997a) Preparing for presymptomatic DNA testing for early onset Alzheimer's disease/cerebral haemorrhage and hereditary Pick disease. *Journal of Medical Genetics* **34**:63–72.

Tibben A, Timman R, Bannick EC *et al.* (1997b) Three-year follow-up after presymptomatic testing for Huntington's disease in tested individuals and partners. *Health Psychology* **16**:30–35.

Triggs-Raine BL, Feigenbaum ASJ, Natowicz M *et al.* (1990) Screening for carriers of Tay-Sachs disease among Ashkenazi Jews: a comparison of DNA-based and enzyme-based tests. *New England Journal of Medicine* **323**:6–12.

Verlinsky Y, Ginsberg N, Lifchez A *et al.* (1990) Analysis of the first polar body: preconception genetic diagnosis. *Human Reproduction* **5**:826–829.

Wachbroit R (1998) The question not asked: the challenge of pleitropic genetic tests. *Kennedy Institute of Ethics Journal* **8**:131–144.

Wertz DC, Fanos JH and Reilly PR (1994) Genetic testing for children and adolescents: who decides? *Journal of the American Medical Association* **272**:875–881.

Wiggins S, Whyte P, Huggins M *et al.* (1992) The psychological consequences of predictive testing for Huntington's disease. *New England Journal of Medicine* **327**:1401–1405.

Wilfond BS and Nolan K (1993) National policy development for the clinical application of genetic diagnostic technologies: lessons from cystic fibrosis. *Journal of the American Medical Association* **270**:2948–2954.

Wolf SM (1995) Beyond 'genetic discrimination': toward the broader harm of geneticism. *Journal of Law and Medical Ethics* **23**:345–353.

Yesley MS (1997) Genetic privacy, discrimination, and social policy: challenges and dilemmas. *Microbial Comparative Genomics* **2**:19–35.

4

To Tell or Not to Tell? The Problem of Medically Unexplained Symptoms

Susan Wessely

ABSTRACT

This essay considers the case of medically unexplained symptoms using two clinical examples: one the problem of hysteria, the other of chronic fatigue syndrome (CFS). I suggest that in both cases doctors' and patients' views on aetiology, diagnosis and treatment are likely to differ. A stark exposition to the patient of the views of most neurologists on the nature of these illnesses is likely to lead to a breakdown of the doctor–patient relationship, and the loss of any chance of instituting meaningful therapy. Instead, patients are more likely to get better when provided with satisfactory explanations for their symptoms—scientifically, culturally and symbolically. I argue that it is the duty of the neurologist first to question his or her underlying assumptions about these illnesses, second to provide a diagnosis acceptable to both scientific rigour and the patients' own views of their illness, and third to use this diagnosis in a constructive fashion. CFS can provide a common starting point for this exploration, and avoids the conflict of diagnosis which commonly occurs. Symptoms believed to be of hysterical origin are more challenging to the neurologist. However, the arguments against an exclusively psychogenic view of any particular symptom are compelling, and permit the neurologist to avoid a confrontation with the patient from which neither party will emerge the winner. Instead a pragmatic approach to treatment which sidesteps the question of aetiology is to be preferred. The aim of the clinical consultation is to help the patient improve—to accept responsibility for recovery without imparting blame or guilt.

INTRODUCTION: THE CONUNDRUM

It is a situation familiar to all clinical neurologists. You have been referred a patient who cannot walk. You have carried out all the examinations, done all the tests. Nothing at all is abnormal. You can find no reason for the patient's

41

disability. You tell the patient that all the tests are normal, and that 'The good news is that you don't have multiple sclerosis'. 'So', replies the patient, 'what is wrong with me?'. What do you say?

Or imagine another scenario. A patient is referred with complaints of fatigue, weakness, memory failure and so on. Again, all tests show nothing. You observe that muscle power is normal, and after a difficult one-hour interview you are fairly convinced that the patient's memory and concentration are the equal of your own. You note a strong previous history of depression, and that in addition to the complaints of easy physical and mental fatigability, the patient also has low mood and sleep disturbance. However, before you can mention the word depression, and indeed before you even carried out your clinical examination, the patient has made it perfectly clear that he is convinced the problem is myalgic encephalomyelitis (ME), otherwise known as CFS.[1] Now your hour is up. The patient looks at you with a mixture of expectancy and mistrust—'Well, doctor, is it ME?', or perhaps 'Doctor, you do believe in ME, don't you?'. What do you reply?

WHAT DO NEUROLOGISTS SAY?

What are the alternatives? Let us begin with the first scenario. What is the diagnosis? If we turn to the latest edition of International Classification of Diseases (ICD-10), or any of the classificatory systems, there seems little doubt this is going to be a case of hysteria, or conversion disorder as we now prefer to call it. So the simplest solution is to tell the patient that this is the problem.

What do neurologists actually do? Mace and Trimble (1991) surveyed British neurologists and showed that they hedged their bets. Although all admitted to seeing patients with non-organic symptoms (how could they not?) 29% said they never used the term hysteria, and another 18% said they used it 'informally', by which they meant in conversation with their colleagues. It is not clear how many would have chosen to use the word in front of the patient (as opposed to in a letter to the GP) but one suspects that it would be very few. Instead, words like 'functional' or 'psychogenic' were frequently used. However, many other terms—supratentorial, neurotic, malingering, psychosomatic, hypochondriasis, conversion, somatoform and so on—were encountered as well.

We can conclude firstly that neurologists rarely use the term hysteria in front of a patient, and secondly that they are inconsistent in what they do say, even to the GP. Quite what they say to the patient remains unclear, but a similar range of euphemisms can be confidently expected.

[1] Myalgic encephalomyelitis' or ME is the popular term for what doctors now call chronic fatigue syndrome (CFS), an operationally defined condition of severe mental and physical fatigability, accompanied by other somatic symptoms, and without conventional medical explanation. The nearest equivalent for ME in the United States would be CFIDS, short for 'chronic fatigue immune dysfunction syndrome'. For a full discussion of the medical, social, cultural and historical background to the fatigue syndromes please see: Wessely S, Hotopf M, Sharpe M 1998 *Chronic Fatigue and its Syndromes*. Oxford: Oxford University Press.

With regard to the second scenario—the patient who confidently states that the problem is ME—I have never seen a survey of the views of practising neurologists, but I have spent plenty of time with them discussing the problem. There has been some change of views over the years, but the conventional neurological view has been often expressed in the literature, and indicates a profound scepticism about the concept of 'myalgic encephalomyelitis'. This scepticism takes several forms. I am unaware of a single neurologist who accepts that the term encephalomyelitis is appropriate for this group of patients, since there is no evidence of an encephalomyelitic process. However, even if one abandons the term ME, and employs the more appropriate one of chronic fatigue syndrome (CFS), it is clear that difficulties remain. One or two neurologists will accept the concept that symptoms result from a primary disorder of muscle, at least in a subgroup, but the majority opinion is that fatigue is of central origin. I suspect that most neurologists remain to be convinced of the role of neuropathological factors, certainly as a cause of long-term disability, and a few continue to harbour very strong sceptical views about the entire subject. A recent survey of general practitioners suggested that, whereas most recognize the illness, most also see it as essentially a psychological problem, or at best as a combination of psychological and neuropathological factors (Campion, personal communication).

There can be little doubt that these views are explicitly not shared by the patient who stands his ground and insists that his problem is 'ME'. It would be tedious to enumerate all the studies that show that one of the characteristics of patients referred to hospital with a label of 'ME' is their strength of conviction that their problems are physical in nature, and that psychological factors play either no role at all, or at best are secondary phenomena ('I may be depressed, but it is because of all the difficulties my illness has caused'). Instead, a common complaint is that psychological problems, when they exist at all, are actually the result of the reluctance doctors show in accepting the physical reality of the patient's illness. This strength of conviction is not found in subjects fulfilling criteria for CFS in the community or in primary care (Euba *et al.*, 1996), but it remains a defining characteristic of patients seen in specialist clinics, who are the subject of this essay.

I have little experience of formal writings on ethics, and qualified from a UK medical school before ethics teaching was a part of the curriculum. Nevertheless, it seems clear that one of the principal ethical duties of the doctor is to tell the truth (Higgs, 1994). Thus, one can argue, with impeccable logic, that it is the duty of the doctor to tell the patient the truth as the doctor sees it. In the first scenario this would involve a simple statement—'Madam, your illness is called hysteria'. In the second scenario, telling the truth, as it appears to the average neurologist, would involve a statement along the lines of 'You do not have ME, you may have something called CFS, but even then I do not believe your problems are neurological, and I think you are depressed'. A neurologist who has kept up with modern psychiatric terminology (no mean accomplishment) might add 'I know you think it is a physical problem, but you are somatizing your psychological distress'. Some readers of this essay, particularly non-neurologists, may passionately disagree that this is the 'truth', but my point is that the above statements accurately reflect the honestly held convictions of many of the specialists to whom this essay is addressed, and that honourable doctors who believe firmly in telling it 'as it is' may find themselves making statements in these terms.

TO DO NO HARM

But what about that other ethical duty 'first, do no harm?'. Could the perceived truth be harmful? Let us start with the patient with hysteria in the first scenario. As far as I am aware, discussions of this issue in the medical ethics literature are largely restricted to the very different scenario of the patient with cancer. I do not think that we can extrapolate from the debate on that issue to the question of whether or not to tell a patient that he or she has a hysterical condition. The word 'hysteria' comes with considerable bag and baggage. It was once seen as a bona fide neurological diagnosis (i.e. a physical illness), but Freud and his followers long since ended that. Psychiatrists may consider it a bona fide psychiatric disorder (hence its continued place in the psychiatric lexicons), but patients assuredly do not. 'Hysteria', 'hysterical' and 'histrionic' are all used interchangeably, and all are unmistakably terms of abuse. 'So it is all in my mind, is it doctor?' says the patient threateningly. The correct answer from our truth-telling neurologist would of course be 'yes', followed by a plaintive 'but psychiatric disorders really are genuine illnesses', but by that time the doctor may well be addressing an empty room, since the patient will have left in disgust.

Our ME patient will react with even more ire. Although there is little evidence to suggest that doctors frequently diagnose hysteria in a patient presenting with severe fatigability, there is plenty to suggest that diagnoses such as depression are commonly made. Depression is, after all, very common amongst chronically fatigued populations (David, 1991). However, whereas most readers of this volume probably consider depression to be a legitimate diagnosis without moral overtones, this view is not shared by those who attribute their symptoms to ME (Wessely, 1994). A recent survey of members of an ME support group showed they did not distinguish between malingering and psychiatric illness, concluding that 'it was assumed that anyone with depression wanted to be ill and taken care of by others' (Ax *et al.*, 1997). Hence the consequences of introducing any psychiatric label are much the same as calling someone hysterical or work shy. I possess several large box files of cuttings from the media and self-help literature in which such scenarios are recounted, followed by passionate denunciations of the doctor for his or her ignorance, cruelty, stupidity, or all of these. Particularly alarming are the many media reports of patients who took their own life, and whose relatives blame not depression, but being told by the doctor it was depression.

Does this matter? If the aim of the neurologist is the simple one of ensuring that he or she does not have to see the patient again, then such an interchange will have achieved the desired effect. However, one trusts that is not the intention. Unfortunately, because patients rarely return to a doctor who they feel is denigrating or discredits their illness experience, whether intentionally or not, that will be the result. This does matter. An essential opportunity for engaging the patient in treatment is lost. Patient satisfaction and functional outcome go together (Woodley *et al.*, 1978). Instead, a disillusioned patient may now turn to the alternative therapists, where the patient can be guaranteed an explanation in keeping with his or her own views of illness, but always at a price. That price also rarely covers any treatment of proven efficacy. The patient will conclude that conventional doctors do not understand, and an ever present polarization between doctor and patient will be reinforced. Also reinforced will be simplistic notions of body and mind: the patient's view that he has a disease solely of the former will now be held with even more conviction, whilst the doctor's suspicion of the key role of the latter may also be confirmed by the vehemence of the patient's response. David Mant has pointed out this Catch 22—the more the patient denies psychosocial causation, the more the doctor suspects it is present (Mant, 1994). Hence if we accept that the 'physician–patient relationship should be ethically sound and therapeutically effective' (Brody, 1994), then one can see many ways in which a physician can achieve the former but only at the cost of the latter.

It is for these reasons that my colleague Tony David (1991) called hysteria the 'H word' —the diagnosis that dare not speak its name. It is not, incidentally, a diagnosis that is disappearing; despite frequent obituaries and plaintive cries of 'where has all the hysteria gone?', studies suggest that it is indeed a tough old bird that has continued to 'outlive its obituarists' (Lewis, 1975; Micale, 1993), and continues to make up about 1% of neurological admissions (Marsden, 1986). It is still around but never spoken about, at least not to the patient. 'A diagnosis which cannot be made face to face with the sufferer and which condemns him to a lifetime of chronic non-recovery if only to prove the doctor wrong is both ethically and strategically wrong' (David, 1993).

WHAT HAPPENS NEXT?

Tony David's last point is crucial. Many satirical news quizzes have sections titled 'What happened next?'. I have often contemplated replaying videos of standard consultations between consultants and patients with ME and asking a similar question. Does anyone seriously consider that the consultant who (and, just like in the quizzes, I add 'allegedly', since no one knows what was actually said) told a medical conference that ME does not exist (Steincamp, 1989) expected his patients to immediately abandon their symptoms and return to work when he shared that information with them? The opposite is more likely. Nortin Hadler (1996) has outlined the dilemma—to get well in these circumstances is to abandon veracity. Patients will be more inclined to get better when they are provided with satisfactory explanations for their problems (Brody, 1994). 'Satisfactory', from the patient's point of view, means not satisfactory in a narrow scientific sense, but satisfactory from a symbolic or even metaphorical perspective (Coulehan, 1991; Kirmayer, 1993; Butler and Rollnick, 1996). Explanations that are not acceptable are not simply discarded; the patient may embark on a mission actively to prove them false.

Another problem, particularly with the modern ME patient, reflects the changing nature of the doctor–patient consultation and the rise of consumerism in general. Patients with hysteria are individuals. Their symptoms are held as individuals, and they rarely, if ever, make common cause with other patients in similar predicaments. This is not always the case with ME. Whether one regards this with approval or irritation (Shorter, 1995), the rise of political pressure groups acting on behalf of patients who believe they have ME is indisputable and awaits its proper analysis. One of the consequences is that patients now have access to alternative sources of information. I have a particular fascination with the history of neurasthenia, the Victorian illness of profound exhaustion which I think is now accepted as the precursor of CFS/ME. The parallels between neurasthenia and CFS are many and inescapable (Wessely, 1996). However, although disputes between doctors about the nature and treatment of neurasthenia were, if anything, more frequent and bitter than modern exchanges on the subject, those between doctors and patients were not. Mistrust and disbelief were certainly present, but they are to be found more in private accounts and coded fictions—the diary of Anne James, sister of William and Henry, the novels of Virginia Woolf and Charlotte Perkins Gilman, and others. What is lacking is the very public confrontation between the patient and the profession that is so striking in the modern discourse on ME. I wonder if the prestige of the Victorian doctor, and conversely the lack of power of the Victorian patient, was such as to make such exchanges difficult. Now all has changed. The modern patient receives information from many sources (Cooper, 1997), can and will go to alternative practitioners if unsatisfied with the conventional physician, and can and often does express dissatisfaction, both in public and with passion. For that reason sociologists have argued that the label of ME has itself come to serve as a symbol for the 'usurpation of power from doctors to patients' (Cooper, 1997). This finds a ready audience with the modern media, fitting as it does a general anti-professional and pro-patient agenda (MacLean and Wessely, 1994).

A DIFFERENT TRUTH?

I hope that I have now convinced the reader that there are insuperable objections to the neurologist 'telling it as he sees it'. The loser is the patient, who will be denied a chance of receiving effective treatment, will be less likely to engage in such treatments at a later date, and will be more likely to shift allegiance to those who are less in a position to help. So is there an alternative?

Let us begin by considering whether or not our conventional neurologist is correct in his or her basic assumptions in the first place. In the first scenario, the case of hysteria, it is difficult to see how one can legitimately expect any major shift in professional views. There seems, however, be more room for change in the ME scenario. I have, for the purpose of this chapter, assumed that the conventional neurological opinion is that CFS is not a neuromuscular disorder and that psychological factors are relevant. The former is almost certainly correct. The latter remains more controversial, but seems to be true in terms of prognosis and/or planning treatment. However, does this mean that physical factors are unimportant? It does not. A brief consideration of the evidence, much of it accumulated in the last two or three years, suggests otherwise. This literature is reviewed in the recent report of the three Royal Colleges (Anon, 1996) and shows that there is compelling evidence that certain infections can trigger CFS. It also shows an increasing body of knowledge that suggests that reproducible abnormalities exist in the hypothalamic–pituitary axis, even if there is no consensus about their interpretation. Others may point to other areas.

Thus honest neurologists now no longer have to make the stark choice between the physical and the psychological. Some might argue that they never have—'this antithesis between "organic" and "functional" disease-states still lingers at the bedside and in medical literature though it is transparently false and has been abandoned long since by all contemplative minds' (Kinnier Wilson, 1940). Doctors like myself with dual qualifications in medicine and psychiatry, and who work in the general hospital, never tire of emphasizing the essential integrity and indivisibility of mind and body, usually ending with impassioned pleas for an end to Cartesian dualism. The fact that we continue to write such pieces testifies to their lack of effect. We live in a dualistic world. Medical students often begin their studies with a non-dualistic concept of the body, which might even be called 'holistic' had the word not been so debased by those professing to practise that kind of medicine. It is striking, and saddening, that they usually leave medical school with a firm Cartesian view, one which, unless they stray into general practice, remains essentially unchanged for the rest of their career. Most of the doctors who research CFS are essentially dualistic, often brutally so. Exceptions, such as the joint immunological and psychiatric team based at Sydney (Wilson *et al.*, 1994) are notable by virtue of their rarity. Patients are also dualistic, not necessarily in their daily lives, but more so when they become sick, and again when they appear in an ME clinic. Hence it is tempting to make a plea for the doctor to make a similarly impassioned speech about the futility of separating mind and body, and the need to see every problem on a holistic basis. In my experience of an ME clinic such attempts are rarely convincing, if not to the doctors, then certainly not to the patient, who usually sees this as a thinly disguised effort to return to the psychological agenda. In the same way, the term 'psychosomatic', which ought to be acceptable in this context (affording equal prominence to psyche and soma) in practice is viewed, correctly, as another addition to the neurologists' non-organic thesaurus (Mace and Trimble, 1991)

I believe that there is convincing evidence of physical precipitants for CFS, and that a physician can now, without committing scientific perjury, share these with the patient. I accept that 'the physician engages in a fundamental fraud if the story offered to explain the illness is not congruent with appropriate scientific thought' (Brody, 1994), a situation all too common in this field. However, I believe that no fraud is being committed in the above narrative and that no ethical imperatives are being breached. On the other hand, by avoiding confrontation, the ethical duty of beneficence is being achieved.

PATIENTS MUST HAVE A DIAGNOSIS

Several studies that concentrate on the views of sufferers confirm that the act of diagnosis is central to the experience of CFS (Ware, 1992; Woodward *et al.*, 1995; Cooper, 1997). Without it the patient feels stigmatized, overlooked and ignored. Worse, the lack of a diagnosis of CFS usually means an alternative diagnosis drawn from the psychiatric section of ICD-10. With the diagnosis comes relief, credibility and acceptance. Some quotes from media articles capture the paradox: 'The day Nomi Antelman learned she had an incurable disease, she rejoiced' (Ames, 1985). Another sufferer was first told she had a virus that would go away. Later this optimistic prognosis was altered, as she learnt she had ME which would, in her own words, take away her independence, regress her to being a baby and in which progress would be minimal. She 'felt fantastic' (Forna, 1987). For another, even if the prognosis was uncertain 'the mental relief was phenomenal' (Brodie, 1988).

Any management strategy that wishes to combine ethics and efficacy must therefore take account of this. Even in general practice we know that patients given a firm diagnosis for non-specific symptoms have a better outcome than those patients randomly allocated to consultations in which uncertainty was expressed (Thomas, 1978). Patients must leave the consultation with a firm diagnosis, otherwise they will be unable to organize their dealings with family, friends and work, let alone consider how to get better. If you do not give them a diagnosis, someone else will. However, it is the ethical duty of the neurologist to avoid the 'contest of diagnosis' (Hadler, 1996) from which neither side will emerge the winner.

PATIENTS WHO SAY THEY HAVE CFS MAY BE RIGHT

The diagnosis must be acceptable to both doctor and patient. One that satisfies the former but not the latter may be ethical, but it will not be effective. I have outlined all the reasons why telling a patient who presents already convinced of the nature of the problem (in this case that they have ME, but for ME substitute any number of other labels) that they are wrong is only acceptable in one situation—when there is a clear-cut, alternative, unambiguous diagnosis, preferably one requiring treatment. Most physicians who are interested in this subject can recount stories of patients with recognized physical disorders which were missed and mislabelled as CFS (Gray *et al.*, 1992; Hurel *et al.*, 1995; Mesch *et al.*, 1996) The list of possible medical causes of CFS is long, but in practice, excluding alternative diagnoses, is relatively straightforward (Matthews *et al.*, 1991).

In all other circumstances it is ruinous to the doctor–patient relationship to tell patients that not only are they wrong, but that the alternative label is one that is totally unacceptable to them—a psychological problem. So why do it? Instead it seems to this author that the only sensible option is to concur. This is ethical: CFS is an operational diagnosis, and if someone fulfils the appropriate criteria, then that is what they have.

After all, how valid are the alternatives? Psychiatric diagnoses have a similar status to CFS: both employ operational criteria and both lack external validation. As Tony Komaroff (1993) elegantly expresses it 'One problem is that CFS is defined by a group of symptoms, without any objective abnormalities on physical examination or laboratory testing that readily establish the diagnosis. Another problem is that the same is true of depression and somatization disorder'. The attempt to replace a solely physical model with an equally monolithic psychogenic explanation is not only doomed to failure, it is also misguided; finally it is, as I shall show in the next section, unnecessary.

DIAGNOSIS IS THE BEGINNING OF THE DIAGNOSTIC PROCESS, AND NOT ITS END

Some doctors will find the previous paragraph difficult to accept. We know that many doctors are reluctant to give a diagnosis of CFS because of their concerns about the impact it might have on the patient's life—indeed, many considered it unethical to do so (Woodward *et al.*, 1995). Such awareness of the possible complications of the diagnosis, and of the dangers of labelling, is both realistic and accurate (Finestone, 1997), most particularly in children (Plioplys, 1997). Given this concern, giving a patient a label that implies both a chronic incurable condition, and one which can only be palliated by chronic rest, is in this view, an indefensible action for a health professional. Confirming the existence of a non-existent pathological process, such as encephalomyelitis, only adds to the patient's difficulties by denying any prospect of cure except a medical 'breakthrough', always promised and never forthcoming.

To avoid this concern, an ethical consultation should be one in which the diagnosis is the beginning, and not the end, of the process. Indeed, this author frequently begins the consultation with the diagnosis 'I agree, you have CFS—

now what do we do about it?' in order to bypass the difficulties that diagnosis involves. A positive diagnosis of CFS has a place in clinical practice, providing that it is used in a constructive fashion. At present CFS can be of use in clinical practice as a structure for patient understanding and a model for treatment, exactly as described in patients presenting with symptoms suggestive of fibromyalgia or irritable bowel syndrome (Kinnier Wilson, 1940; Goldenberg, 1995; Sharpe *et al.*, 1997).

It is not the place of this essay to outline what happens next. In practice this involves broadening the assessment to take account of all the factors, physical, cognitive, emotional, behavioural and so on, that come together in the final common illness presentation that is CFS. This multidimensional approach has been outlined elsewhere (Sharpe *et al.*, 1997), and has empirical support as a basis for treatment (Sharpe *et al.*, 1996; Deale *et al.*, 1997). There is also evidence to support the particular position adopted in this essay. It is now clear that, in order to improve, patients do not need to, and indeed do not, alter their views that either their problem is ME/CFS or that it began as a physical illness. Instead, improvement only requires a shift in the patient's view on the relative merits of rest and exercise (Deale *et al.*, 1998). Patients with CFS usually believe that rest is the best way of controlling symptoms, and are otherwise relatively powerless to alter the course of the illness (Clements *et al.*, 1997). Disability is related to the presence of catastrophic beliefs about the disastrous effect of activity (Petrie *et al.*, 1995). Effective management involves challenging these assumptions, but not the physical origin of illness (Sharpe *et al.*, 1996; Deale *et al.*, 1997).

DO WE NEED TO TELL ANYTHING AT ALL?

Let us now return to the more difficult scenario, the patient with hysteria. Here a thorough understanding of medical science cannot come to our aid by giving us an entrée into the patient's own illness world. Recent reviews have highlighted the physiological mechanisms underlying symptoms experienced by somatizing patients and hence have helped to lay to rest the spectre of 'all in the mind'[2] (Sharpe and Bass, 1992; White and Moorey, 1997) but it is noticeable that they did not attempt the more difficult task of a similar synthesis for hysterical symptoms. The recent inspired use of neuroimaging to elucidate the neurobiological basis of hysterical symptoms (inhibition by subcortical pathways of the cortical initiation of movement) may give some guidance (Marshall *et al.*, 1997), but this is certainly not the case at present. When the medical ethicist Roger Higgs (1994) writes that 'trust and truth telling are intimately involved' he is implying that trust between doctor and patient can only result from truth telling, and that to do otherwise is an act of deception

---

[2] This begs the question of what exactly an illness that was 'all in the mind' would look like, and if any such condition is conceptually possible. However, this is not the place to enter into a discussion of the mind–body question in Western philosophy.

that will inevitably damage both parties. The hysteria scenario, however, seems to prove the opposite contention—trust between doctor and patient may be better served by not telling the truth.

Given the clear ethical imperative against lying, what can be left? I suggest that the solution is to say little. Is it imperative that the patient be told that the illness is truly 'all in the mind'? I suspect not. In the classic formulation of hysteria the illness arises from the repression of intolerable psychic trauma, which then 're-emerges' as physical loss of function. This steam kettle model of the psyche has notable intellectual origins, and an equally notable lack of empirical validation. Sometimes in extreme conditions, such as wartime, examples can be found, but all too often in civilian medical practice the doctor struggles to find 'something nasty in the woodshed' to explain the dramatic loss of function. Likewise, classic psychiatric teaching, still inspired (if that is the word) by Freud, teaches that only by identifying the cause of the trauma, and by allowing the patient to 'work through it', will the loss of function be corrected. Again, empirical backing for this position is lacking.

Instead, what works in the treatment of hysteria is considerably more prosaic. The treatment of hysterical loss of function is remarkably similar to that of non-hysterical loss of function. In children, recovery occurred rapidly when further investigations were banned and graded exercise was given by physiotherapists (Leslie, 1988). Patients with hysterical paraplegias were told they had 'spinal concussion'; this was followed by directed exercises and constant reinforcement that they would get better. They did (Baker and Silver, 1987). Operant conditioning proved successful in a recent report (Kop *et al.*, 1995). The message seems to be that there is no need to confront the patient with the H word in order to effect recovery.

CONCLUSION

To tell or not to tell? The answer is to tell, but to make sure that what you tell is both accurate and pragmatic. The aim of telling is to help the patient get better. Each doctor will find his or own individual style in deciding what to tell. However, whatever you decide, remember that the goal of telling is to assist patients in assuming responsibility for their recovery but without inducing any guilt or blame for why they became ill in the first place.

REFERENCES

Ames M (1985) Learning to live with incurable virus. *Chicago Tribune* June 9th 1985; Section 5, p. 3.
Anon (1996) *Chronic Fatigue Syndrome: Report of a Committee of the Royal Colleges of Physicians, Psychiatrists and General Practitioners*. London: Royal Colleges of Physicians.
Ax S, Gregg V and Jones D (1997) Chronic fatigue syndrome: sufferers' evaluation of medical support. *Journal of the Royal Society of Medicine* 90:250–254.

Baker J and Silver J (1987) Hysterical paraplegia. *Journal of Neurology, Neurosurgery and Psychiatry* **50**:375–382.

Brodie E (1988) Understanding M.E. *Nursing Times* **84**:48–49.

Brody H (1994) 'My story is broken: can you help me fix it?' Medical ethics and the joint construction of narrative. *Literature and Medicine* **13**:79–92.

Butler C and Rollnick S (1996) Missing the meaning and provoking resistance: a case of myalgic encephalomyelitis. *Family Practice* **13**:106–109.

Clements A, Sharpe M, Simkin S, Borrill J and Hawton K (1997) Chronic fatigue syndrome: a qualitative investigation of patients' beliefs about the illness. *Journal of Psychosomatic Research* **42**:615–624.

Cooper L (1997) Myalgic encephalomyelitis and the medical encounter. *Sociology of Health and Illness* **19**:17–37.

Coulehan J (1991) The word is an instrument of healing. *Literature and Medicine* **10**:111–129.

David A (1993) Camera, lights, action for ME. *British Medical Journal* **307**:688.

David AS (1991) Postviral fatigue syndrome and psychiatry. *British Medical Bulletin* **47**:966–988.

Deale A, Chalder T, Marks I and Wessely S (1997) A randomised controlled trial of cognitive behaviour versus relaxation therapy for chronic fatigue syndrome. *American Journal of Psychiatry* **154**:408–414.

Deale A, Chalder T and Wessely S (1998) Illness beliefs and outcome in chronic fatigue syndrome: is change in causal attribution necessary for clinical improvement? *Journal of Psychosomatic Research* **45**:77–83.

Euba R, Chalder T, Deale A and Wessely S (1996) A comparison of the characteristics of chronic fatigue syndrome in primary and tertiary care. *British Journal of Psychiatry* **168**:121–126.

Finestone AJ (1997) A doctor's dilemma. Is a diagnosis disabling or enabling? *Archives of Internal Medicine* **157**:491–492.

Forna A (1987) A real pain. *Girl About Town* 21st May 1987.

Goldenberg D (1995) Fibromyalgia: why such controversy? *Annals of the Rheumatic Diseases* **54**:3–5.

Gray J, Bridges A and McNeill G (1992) Atrial myxoma: a rare cause of progressive exertional dyspnoea. *Scottish Medical Journal* **37**:186–187.

Hadler NM (1996) If you have to prove you are ill, you can't get well. The object lesson of fibromyalgia. *Spine* **21**:2397–2400.

Higgs R (1994) Truth telling, lying and the doctor-patient relationship. In: *Principles of Health Care Ethics* (ed. R Gillon), pp. 499–509. Chichester: John Wiley.

Hurel S, Abuiasha B, Bayliss P and Harris P (1995) Patients with a self diagnosis of myalgic encephalomyelitis. *British Medical Journal* **311**:329.

Kinnier Wilson S (1940) *Neurology*, Vol. 2. New York: Hafner.

Kirmayer L (1993) Healing and the invention of metaphor: the effectiveness of symbols revisited. *Culture, Medicine and Psychiatry* **17**:161–195.

Komaroff A (1993) Clinical presentation of chronic fatigue syndrome. In: *Chronic Fatigue Syndrome* (eds S Straus, A Kleinman), pp 43–61. Vol. 173. Chichester: John Wiley.

Kop P, van der Heijden H, Hoogduin K and Schaap C (1995) Operant procedures applied to a conversion disorder. *Clinical Psychology and Psychotherapy* **2**:59–66.

Leslie S (1988) Diagnosis and treatment of hysterical conversion reactions. *Archives of Disease in Childhood* **63**:506–511.

Lewis A (1975) The survival of hysteria. *Psychological Medicine* **5**:9–12.

Mant D (1994) Chronic fatigue syndrome. *Lancet* **344**:834–835.

Mace CJ and Trimble MR (1991) 'Hysteria', 'functional' or 'psychogenic'? A survey of British neurologists preferences. *Journal of the Royal Society of Medicine* **84**:471–475.

MacLean G and Wessely S (1994) Professional and popular representations of chronic fatigue syndrome. *British Medical Journal* **308**:776–777.

Marsden C (1986) Hysteria—a neurologist's view. *Psychological Medicine* **16**:277–288.

Marshall J, Halligan P, Fink G, Wade D and Frackowiak R (1997) The functional anatomy of a hysterical paralysis. *Cognition* **64**:B1–B8.

Matthews D, Manu T and Lane T (1991) Evaluation and management of patients with chronic fatigue. *American Journal of Medical Science* **302**:269–277.

Mesch U, Lowenthal R and Colemen D (1996) Lead poisoning masquerading as chronic fatigue syndrome. *Lancet* **347**:1193.

Micale M (1993) On the 'disappearance' of hysteria: a study in the clinical deconstruction of a diagnosis. *Isis* **84**:496–526.

Petrie K, Moss-Morris R and Weinman J (1995) The impact of catastrophic beliefs on functioning in chronic fatigue syndrome. *Journal of Psychosomatic Research* **39**:31–37.

Plioplys A (1997) Chronic fatigue syndrome should not be diagnosed in children. *Pediatrics* **100**:270–271.

Sharpe M and Bass C (1992) Pathophysiological mechanisms in somatization. *International Review of Psychiatry* **4**:81–97.

Sharpe M, Hawton K, Simkin S. *et al.* (1996) Cognitive behaviour therapy for chronic fatigue syndrome; a randomized controlled trial. *British Medical Journal* **312**:22–26.

Sharpe M, Chalder T, Palmer I and Wessely S (1997) Chronic fatigue syndrome: a practical guide to assessment and management. *General Hospital Psychiatry* **19**:195–199.

Shorter E (1995) Sucker-punched again! Physicians meet the disease-of-the-month syndrome. *Journal of Psychosomatic Research* **39**:115–188.

Steincamp J (1989) *Overload: Beating M.E.* London: Fontana, 1989.

Thomas K (1978) The consultation and the therapeutic illusion. *British Medical Journal* **1**:1327–1328.

Ware N (1992) Suffering and the social construction of illness: the delegitimisation of illness experience in chronic fatigue syndrome. *Medical Anthropology Quarterly* **6**:347–361.

Wessely S (1994) Neurasthenia and chronic fatigue: theory and practice in Britain and America. *Transcultural Psychiatry Research Review* **31**:173–209.

Wessely S (1996) Neurasthenia and chronic fatigue. In: Porter R, Berrios G, eds. *The History of Psychiatry* (eds R Porter, G Berrios), pp. 509–532. London: Athlone.

White P and Moorey S (1997) Psychosomatic disorders are not 'all in the mind'. *Journal of Psychosomatic Research* **42**:329–332.

Wilson A, Hickie I, Lloyd A and Wakefield D (1994) The treatment of chronic fatigue syndrome; science and speculation. *American Journal of Medicine* **96**:544–549.

Woodley F, Kane R, Hughes C and Wright D (1978) The effects of doctor-patient communication on satisfaction and outcome of care. *Social Science and Medicine* **12**:123–128.

Woodward R, Broom D and Legge D (1995) Diagnosis in chronic illness: disabling or enabling—the case of chronic fatigue syndrome. *Journal of the Royal Society of Medicine* **88**:325–329.

5

Should the Diagnosis of Alzheimer's Disease Always Be Disclosed?

Robert Howard

ABSTRACT

The doctors and carers of patients with Alzheimer's disease are often hesitant to share the diagnosis with the sufferer, despite evidence that most of us would wish to be told. The approach to breaking this news should be tailored to individual circumstances. There is little merit in communicating complex information to a patient with severe dementia, but in general the arguments for sensitive disclosure of this diagnosis to the sufferer will outweigh the case against. Such disclosure will give the sufferer the opportunity to plan for the future.

INTRODUCTION

The right of an individual patient to know when he or she has been diagnosed with a progressive, irreversible and terminal illness would seem self-evident (Davidson, 1957) and is enshrined in *The Patient's Charter* (Department of Health, 1992). As we shall see, when the diagnosis is Alzheimer's disease (AD), the issue of disclosure is not so clear-cut. Although the ethical and practical arguments for telling AD patients their diagnosis probably outweigh those against (Drickamer and Lachs, 1992; Meyers, 1997), old age psychiatrists and our colleagues in neurology and geriatric medicine do not reveal the diagnosis in the majority of cases.

WHAT CONSTITUTES BEST PRACTICE ON DIAGNOSTIC DISCLOSURE?

The American Psychiatric Association's *Practice Guidelines for the Treatment of Patients with Alzheimer's Disease and Other Dementias of Late Life* (American Psychiatric Association, 1997) provide an important and authoritative guide to optimum physician conduct with AD patients and their carers. At last, guidelines have gone beyond instructions on how to make the diagnosis and extend to how most usefully to communicate information to patients and their families. The guidelines place special emphasis on the importance of establishing and maintaining an alliance with the patient and his family in successful management. The family are a critical (sometimes the only) source of information about the patient; they will be responsible for implementing and monitoring treatment plans in the home, and their attitudes and behaviours have a profound effect on the patient. The psychiatrist has a responsibility to educate the patient and family about the illness and its natural history. An important step in this process is to communicate the diagnosis, but patients vary in their awareness and ability to discuss this, and so an explicit discussion with family members regarding diagnosis, prognosis and options for intervention will often come first. This will help them to recognize current symptoms and anticipate future manifestations of the illness; it also allows education about basic principles of care such as the avoidance of complex instructions and tasks or confrontation with the patient. Most mildly affected patients can discuss the diagnosis at some level, but the guidelines make clear that such discussions must be adapted to the specific concerns and abilities of each patient. The guidelines thus give an unambiguous message about disclosing the diagnosis: you do it, but through involvement with the family and in your dealings with the patient, in a manner which is responsive to his questions and appropriate to his level of understanding.

WHO TELLS?

Disclosing behaviour of physicians involved in the diagnosis and care of patients with AD has been the subject of research study. Rice and Warner (1994) sent questionnaires to 326 UK old age psychiatrists to survey their practice in telling patients the diagnosis at various stages of AD. Although carers were almost invariably informed of the diagnosis, patients with severe dementia were almost never told. In mild dementia about 30%, and in moderate dementia about 55%, of patients were not told their diagnoses. These authors reported a wide range of approaches among old age psychiatrists. Some provided information about diagnosis and prognosis only if the patient specifically requested it, while others suggested imparting the diagnosis gradually over a series of follow-up interviews. Many of the respondents noted that relatives are often very protective of patients and that it is often very easy to fall into collusion with this. The same group of authors (Rice *et al.*, 1997) sent questionnaires to 318 geriatric physicians and again found a wide range of practice on telling patients with AD their diagnosis. In cases of mild dementia, geriatricians seemed to tell fewer carers and more patients what the diagnosis was than did the old age psychiatrists, but otherwise the behaviour of these two groups of doctors was very similar.

WHAT DO CARERS AND PATIENTS WANT?

We know very little about what AD patients want to be told, and the voice of the patient is markedly absent from the literature. A study of cognitively intact patients in primary care, only some of whom were elderly, found that very few of them would not want to know the diagnosis if they developed AD (Erde *et al.*, 1988). In a survey of 100 consecutive family members of AD patients seen in a memory clinic (Maguire *et al.*, 1996), participants were asked whether the patient with AD should be told their diagnosis and whether they themselves would want to be told if they had AD. Eighty-three per cent said that the patient should not be told, but 71% wanted to be told themselves if they developed AD. A paternalistic approach by family members to protect the patient from the harsh reality of their condition together with a reluctance of relatives to deal with the patient's knowledge and subsequent grief were considered to lie behind this inconsistency. A different result was reported by Barnes (1997), who found that only 43% of the carers he questioned would want to have the diagnosis kept from the patient.

THE CASE FOR NOT TELLING

Since it appears to fly in the face of so much that seems self-evident in the ethical and practical treatment and care of AD patients, and so that it does not get lost following a list of the benefits of telling patients their diagnosis, the case against disclosing diagnosis will be put first. The author does not intend to construct a straw man of the case against telling, only to have this blown aside by substantial counter arguments. Rather he hopes that, by considering the negative arguments first, at least some of the principles which underlie them will impress the reader, who may then be slightly less inclined to swallow uncritically all the political correctness and practical appeal of the positive view.

The rationale for withholding information about diagnosis rests on the physician's responsibility to prevent harm (Gillon, 1985). There are situations, for example in some paranoid psychoses, when the practical case for not disclosing diagnosis is overwhelming (Howard, 1993). The strongest and most convincing argument for not telling patients with AD their diagnosis is that the capacity of patients to understand the diagnosis and deal with the implications depends both upon their cognitive function and psychiatric state. Either or both of these variables may be seriously affected by the disease.

Let us deal first with understanding of diagnosis. Some moderately demented patients and almost all with severe AD are incapable of processing and retaining even the most trivial information. What could possibly be the point of conveying information about diagnosis and prognosis in such cases? Even if patients were able to echo the words of the informing physician, would they truly have comprehended and be able to retain the information? Since the only way one could assess the transfer of information in many such cases would be to observe the patient for clear signs of distress and unhappiness, this would not be an easy time for patient, carer or physician.

One logical way to solve this problem would be to identify patients earlier in the course of the illness when understanding is not impaired. Early identification of AD cases using neuropsychological testing to demonstrate subtle deficits might however reveal cases which are still subclinical and one would have to ask whether such aggressive early case-finding would actually be of any benefit or service to patients.

A common fear expressed by carers, perhaps shared by some health care professionals, is that awareness of the diagnosis in insightful patients will precipitate distress or even a severe depressive reaction. Indeed, there are case reports of suicide in AD patients soon after being told their diagnoses (Rohde *et al.*, 1995). The evidence is not strong, however, for such a harmful effect of disclosure in the great majority of cases (Meyers, 1997). Although common sense and clinical experience would suggest that confrontation of cognitive deficit and diagnosis often leads to transient emotional reaction, there is no good evidence of long-term effects. The ability of AD patients to utilize psychological defences such as denial is often intact early in the illness course (Bahro *et al.*, 1995), and neuropsychological deficits such as anosognosia may also help to soften the blow (Michen *et al.*, 1994).

A second argument that is put against disclosure is that, since a diagnosis of AD made during the patient's lifetime can never be made with more confidence than the prefix 'probable' might suggest, unless they have been the victims of a brain biopsy patients should not be burdened with such an uncertain diagnosis. In reality, neuropathological confirmation of AD diagnoses made during life runs at well over 90% and, of the remaining cases, practically all have evidence of some other degenerative dementing process.

Prognosis is so variable between individual AD cases, that it is also sometimes argued that it is better to avoid disclosing information about diagnosis and illness progression because such information may not match with what the patient and carer subsequently experience. While prognostication is imprecise and the nature of cognitive, behavioural and functional impairments as well as their tempo and severity are all variable, there can be little doubt that both patients and their carers cope better with difficulties they have been prepared for and warned to expect.

THE CASE FOR TELLING

We have already briefly considered the issue of a person's right to have explained to them what is wrong, and to come to terms with their diagnosis by submission, reconciliation or protest, but at least in the dignity of knowledge. There are of course also some extremely practical advantages to disclosure of diagnosis in AD. To accept or forgo those treatments, the advent of which is certainly upon us (Rogers *et al.*, 1996), specifically for the symptoms of AD and interventions affecting loss of function and independence, patients with AD will want to be given the best available information about their condition so that their decisions can be as informed as possible. Individuals may also wish to formulate advance directives while they are still competent to do so. Knowledge of diagnosis in such a competent patient will allow him to make financial arrangements, settle his personal affairs and seek further medical advice—maybe even a second opinion if the news is too difficult to believe.

Since the effective treatments available for cognitive deficit in AD are palliative and may only work during a short period of illness progression, a huge research effort can be expected by the pharmaceutical companies keen to extend this modest success to find a 'cure' for the condition. Fully informed patients can apprise their surrogates of their wishes concerning subsequent participation in medical research. The line between ethical and exploitative research on demented subjects is a fine one, and there are some interesting research indicators that decisions made by surrogates are not always accurate. In a nursing home setting, 78 out of 169 surrogates refused consent to involvement of patients in a simple study of the use of urinary catheters (Warren *et al.*, 1986). Disturbingly, even though 55 surrogates said that they believed the patient would have refused consent to the study, 17 of these surrogates consented to involvement anyway.

There is another argument in favour of telling which involves the health and safety of us all. If you want to stop AD patients from using their cars, then it is difficult to do this without disclosing the diagnosis. Most available evidence suggests that even mild dementia impairs driving performance (Hunt *et al.*, 1993), but that AD patients continue to drive (Carr *et al.*, 1990; Gilley *et al.*, 1991). There is no consensus concerning the threshold at which AD patients should be stopped from driving. Since there do not seem to be any features of the condition which are clearly predictive of either safety or dangerousness behind the wheel, but the illness is predictably progressive, the author believes that all patients with diagnosable AD should be told not to drive. The APA guidelines do not go so far, but recommend that psychiatrists should discuss the risks of driving with all demented patients and their families and that these discussions should be carefully documented in the patient's notes.

THE REALITY OF TELLING AND NOT TELLING

While it is clear in principle that those patients with AD who can comprehend the diagnosis, wish to be told it and are psychologically prepared and supported to cope with the information should be told that they have the illness, the situation in the clinic is rarely like this. Because of delays in detection of deficit and referral to a physician who is competent and confident to make the diagnosis, probably at least one half of patients seen by old age psychiatrists for assessment will not understand or remember for more than a few seconds any information they are given about diagnosis. Among the remainder, while each case must be handled on an individual basis, there is an element of urgency to communicate information about diagnosis while that information may still be of practical use to the sufferer. In such cases the presence or absence of insight into deficit is an important indicator of how the news should be conveyed. Patients with insight retention often suspect or know the worst already. They may harbour the fantasy that decline into mute, helpless dependence is only weeks or months away and so disclosure of diagnosis with frank discussion of likely prognosis may come as something of a relief to them. Although insightful patients are considered to be most at risk of deliberate self-harm after disclosure of diagnosis, suicide in this group is extremely rare and probably no more common than in patients in the early stages of many disabling disorders. The patient's ability to absorb and cope with distressing information and the support from family or other sources of care should be assessed as part of the diagnostic evaluation. The timing and method of telling can be tailored in the light of these factors. It is unacceptable to leave the job of diagnostic disclosure to the families of such patients.

For the insightless patient who is able to understand and remember what you have told him, yet through neuropsychological deficit cannot recognize in himself what is being disclosed, in uncomplicated cases the physician has a duty to tell once. There is no evidence to suggest that repeatedly rubbing the sufferer's nose in his diagnosis will help him to develop insight. This situation can, however, be complicated by situations such as the patient continuing to drive against medical advice. In such cases the diagnosis does need to be repeated, not in any kind of attempt to help the patient accept his diagnosis, but rather to reinforce his continuing responsibilities to society.

In those patients who are severely affected by the illness, there seems little point in telling them their diagnosis just because one supports the principle of telling. In each case the sufferer's need for information and communication should be assessed, even if a handshake or a hug is the only communication that seems to be helpful in the end.

CONCLUSION

While the arguments in favour of disclosing diagnosis in AD trump those against this practice, each case merits individual consideration, making the formulation of blanket guidelines problematic. Telling the diagnosis is certainly harder than not telling for both physicians and informal carers, but the irresistible advance of political correctness and so-called patients' rights groups could have unhelpful consequences. I dread the day I walk onto a dementia care unit to be greeted by an orientation chart that reads 'Today is Wednesday. The Weather is Sunny. The Next Meal is Breakfast. You All Have Alzheimer's Disease'.

REFERENCES

American Psychiatric Association (1997) Practice guidelines for the treatment of patients with Alzheimer's disease and other dementias of late life. *American Journal of Psychiatry* **154(5)**:Suppl. 1–39.

Bahro M, Silber E and Sunderland R (1995) How do patients with Alzheimer's disease cope with illness? A clinical experience report. *Journal of the American Geriatric Society* **43**:41–46.

Barnes RC (1997) Telling the diagnosis to patients with Alzheimer's disease. *British Medical Journal* **314**:375–376.

Carr D, Jackson T and Alquire P (1990) Characteristics of an elderly driving population referred to a geriatric assessment centre. *Journal of the American Geriatric Society* **38**:1145–1150.

Davidson M (1957) *Medical Ethics—A Guide to Students and Practitioners.* London: Lloyd-Luke.

Department of Health (1992) *The Patient's Charter.* London: DoH.

Drickamer MA and Lachs MS (1992) Should patients with Alzheimer's disease be told their diagnosis? *New England Journal of Medicine* **326**:947–951.

Erde EL, Nadal EC and Scholl TO (1988) On truth telling and the diagnosis of Alzheimer's disease. *Journal of Family Practice* **26**:401–406.

Gilley DW, Wilson RS, Bennett DA, Stebbings GT, Bernard BA, Whalen ME and Fox JH (1991) Cessation of driving and unsafe motor operation by dementia patients. *Archives of Internal Medicine* **151**:941–946.

Gillon R (1985) Telling the truth and medical ethics. *British Medical Journal* **291**:1556–1557.

Howard R (1993) Insight and honesty. *British Medical Journal* **306**:764.

Hunt L, Morris JC, Edwards D and Wilson BA (1993) Driving performance in persons with mild senile dementia of the Alzheimer type. *Journal of the American Geriatric Society* **41**:747–753.

Maguire CP, Kirby M, Coen R, Coakley D, Lawlor BA and O'Neill D (1996) Family members' attitudes toward telling the patient with Alzheimer's disease their diagnosis. *British Medical Journal* **313**:529–530.

Meyers BS (1997) Telling patients they have Alzheimer's disease. *British Medical Journal* **341**:321–322.

Michen A, Deweer B, Pitlon B, Agid Y and Dubois B (1994) Relation of anosognosia to frontal lobe dysfunction in Alzheimer's disease. *Journal of Neurology, Neurosurgery and Psychiatry* **57**:805–809.

Rice K and Warner N (1994) Breaking the bad news: What do psychiatrists tell patients with dementia about their illness? *International Journal of Geriatric Psychiatry* **9**:467–471.

Rice K, Warner N, Tye T and Bayer A (1997) Geriatricians' and psychiatrists' practice differs. *British Medical Journal* **314**:376.

Rogers SL, Friedhoff LT, Apter JT *et al.* (1996) The efficacy and safety of donepezil in patients with Alzheimer's disease: Results of a US multicentre, randomized, double-blind, placebo-controlled trial. *Dementia* **7**:293–303.

Rohde K, Peskind ER and Raskind MA (1995) Suicide in two patients with Alzheimer's disease. *Journal of the American Geriatric Society* **43**:187–189.

Warren JW, Sobal J and Tenney JH (1986) Informed consent by proxy: An issue in research with elderly patients. *New England Journal of Medicine* **315**:1124–1128.

6

When, If Ever, Should Confidentiality Be Set Aside?

Jessica Wilen Berg

ABSTRACT

Physicians need to understand the ethical basis for confidentiality protection as well as be familiar with the general categories of exceptions. This essay addresses the situations when physicians are legally permitted, and sometimes legally required, to breach patient confidentiality. Although there is a variety of legal and ethical reasons put forward for confidentiality, no theory provides complete protection from disclosure, and each allows for exceptions based on a balancing of the interests promoted by confidentiality versus the interests promoted by disclosure. There are four general areas in which US law has determined that balance may favour disclosure, and each is discussed separately: public health; public safety; protection of vulnerable persons; and statistical registries.

INTRODUCTION

A young woman appears at a public health clinic and tests positive for HIV, the virus that causes AIDS. Within the next few months a number of other women show up, all testing positive. When asked about sexual partners, each provides a description of the same young man, using various aliases, who cannot be located by health officials. The man, Nushawn Williams, is eventually traced to a prison in New York City. Before health officials finally obtain a court order authorizing disclosure of his name and HIV status, he is estimated to have infected at least 13 people. (Davis, 1997)

When should confidentiality be set aside? In order to answer this question, one must examine the rationale underlying confidentiality in the medical setting. Despite the overt general acceptance of confidentiality within the medical community, it has never functioned as an absolute bar to disclosure (Gellman, 1984). First, legal and ethical protections may be waived. No breach occurs when a patient has authorized disclosure. For example, a patient might request that a physician share information on health care matters with the patient's spouse or a close friend. Second, when the patient is incompetent, certain individuals may be legally authorized to receive information that would otherwise be confidential. Thus, surrogates or health care guardians have a right to their ward's medical information, and parents generally have a right to their children's medical information.[1] Third, although there are a number of different bases for confidentiality, no theory provides complete protection from disclosure, and each allows for exceptions based on a balancing of the interests promoted by confidentiality versus the interests promoted by disclosure. The following sections examine the ethical and legal rationale underlying protection of confidentiality in the medical setting and identify four general areas in which US law has determined that balance may favour disclosure.[2]

BASIS FOR CONFIDENTIALITY

It is quite common to talk about the physician's duty to keep information confidential. The concept of confidentiality dates back at least to the earliest codes of medical ethics. The Hippocratic Oath, for example, requires the physician to promise that 'What I may see or hear in the course of the treatment or even outside of the treatment in regard to the life of men, which on no account one must spread abroad, I will keep to myself holding such things shameful to be spoken about' (Temkin and Temkin, 1967). More recent ethical codes also include statements on confidentiality. The World Medical Organization's *Declaration of Geneva* and the International Code of Medical Ethics both admonish the physician to maintain confidentiality even after the patient's death (Friedland, 1994). The American Medical Association's (AMA's) *Code of Medical Ethics* states that 'the information disclosed to the physician during the course of the relationship between the physician and patient is confidential to the greatest possible degree' (AMA Opinion 5.05, 1996). But unlike the early codes, the AMA's requirement immediately recognizes a number of exceptions to confidentiality 'justified by overriding social considerations'.

The rationale underlying the ethical theories is essentially a practical, or consequential one: 'The patient should feel free to make a full disclosure of information to the physician in order that the physician may most effectively provide needed services' (AMA Opinion 5.05, 1996). Confidentiality is thus thought to be a necessary requirement of the patient–physician relationship. Without assurances of privacy, patients may be less likely to disclose information pertinent to their medical care. For example, because of the high risk of discrimination, patients may be unwilling to disclose HIV status if they fear disclosure. As a result, physicians will be unable to provide appropriate treatment.

[1] The issue of confidentiality in the context of minor patients is beyond the scope of this chapter.
[2] All references in this chapter refer to US federal and state laws.

In addition to weighing the costs and benefits of protecting privacy, there may also be other bases for confidentiality protections. For example, privacy and confidentiality may have value in and of themselves, regardless of the practical effects of protections or lack of protections. Whether based on a concern about the consequences of disclosure or the inherent value of privacy, a general requirement of confidentiality is applied to medical practice. However, exceptions to this general rule apply when the cost of maintaining confidences is outweighed by the harm to others. As the Williams case described at the beginning of this chapter makes clear, other individuals may have a valid interest in obtaining otherwise confidential medical information about a patient.[3]

The ethical requirements of confidentiality are not easily separated from the legal framework. The AMA Code, for example, clearly defers to the law. At least one commentator argues that the AMA abrogates its responsibility to maintain confidentiality by failing to articulate the ethical exceptions separately from the legal requirements, even if the result would be that physicians must disobey the law to comply with ethics (McConnell, 1994). Although I will focus below on the US laws that carve out exceptions, this should not be taken to imply that the scope of the ethical duty to maintain confidentiality matches exactly the scope of the legal requirements. Disclosure is only ethical when the law in question correctly balances the physician's duty to his or her patient versus the physician's duty to others who may be harmed by the lack of disclosure.

At the outset it is important to distinguish between legal protections for confidentiality and legal privileges. Privileges are evidentiary protections that function in the context of litigation. In other words, they prevent certain information from being used as evidence in a legal case. Historically, information disclosed by a patient to a physician could not be disclosed by the physician in the course of legal proceedings without the patient's permission, with few exceptions. Thus, a physician could not be forced to reveal patient confidences in the courtroom. Nowadays most states have dispensed with the patient–physician privilege (Smith, 1986). The one exception to this is the psychotherapist–patient privilege, which remains viable.

Legal protections of confidentiality take up where privileges leave off. There are a number of different legal bases for imposing confidentiality requirements on physicians. One is derived from contract law. This theory has its premise in the notion that the covenant between physician and patient includes an implied promise not to reveal information gained as part of the treatment relationship (Horne v. Patton, 1973). Although there is certainly some expectation of confidentiality on the part of the patient, it is unclear whether this is sufficient to give rise to a contractual duty. Moreover, implied contracts must be proven—they do not automatically give rise to specific duties. As a result, patients are not necessarily guaranteed confidentiality.

---

[3]A recent study shows that many HIV+ individuals do not disclose their status to sexual partners (Stein *et al.*, 1998).

A second legal basis for confidentiality is fiduciary theory, which provides a default rule for maintaining confidentiality. Instead of requiring a patient to demonstrate an implied contract in each case, the physician would have to challenge the presumption of confidentiality by showing the absence of a fiduciary (e.g., patient–physician) relationship. Fiduciary theory arose out of contractual relationships in which one party was particularly vulnerable and unable to protect himself against a breach (Scalen, 1991). The traditional cases of agent–principal and trustee–beneficiary have been expanded in recent years to include the patient–physician relationship. In some ways, the fiduciary model fits well—the patient is clearly a vulnerable party. By applying traditional fiduciary principles, the physician is held responsible for maintaining confidentiality of all information entrusted to her by the patient (Restatement, 1958). But physicians do not fit perfectly into the fiduciary model (Rodwin, 1995).

Confidentiality in the traditional fiduciary relationship is not defined as a ban on disclosing information, but rather a duty to use confidential information to the benefit of the vulnerable party. How benefit is interpreted depends on the fiduciary's role. A fiduciary must have a defined role—in the classic agency case it is to promote profit (Frankel, 1983). It is not as easy to ascribe a single responsibility to a physician. Should the focus be on prolonging life? Minimizing suffering? Curing disease? The requirement of confidentiality would only apply if its application furthered the primary obligation of the fiduciary. For example, if the physician's primary role is to prolong life, confidentiality should be breached when the disclosure would serve to prolong life, or the failure to disclose would shorten life. Thus a patient's threat of suicide should be disclosed in order to prevent harm to self. On the other hand, if the primary goal is to minimize suffering, then it is less clear whether a threat of suicide should be disclosed.[4]

Since neither contract nor fiduciary law provides clear guidance for the application of confidentiality, one might look to constitutional and common law privacy principles. There are, in the US, constitutional privacy protections of an individual's home (US Const. Amend. IV), body (Cruzan v. Director, Missouri Dept of Health, 1990), and personal information (US Dept of Justice v. Reporters' Comm., 1989). But personal information is not protected at law in the same way as one's home or bodily integrity is protected. In fact, quite a bit of personal information is not protected at all. For example, it is fairly simple to obtain a person's credit history in contrast to his or her medical history despite the fact that both may be considered highly personal information. One author notes that privacy protections are basically a means to protect other interests such as reputation, avoidance of embarrassment or shame, or discrimination (Murphy, 1996).[5] If so, then protections for confidentiality should function only

[4]This presupposes both that there can be a rational threat of suicide, and that the patient's threat is not a plea for help.
[5]The information in question may not be shameful on its own (e.g. private details of bedroom practices) but may cause shame if revealed to others.

to the extent that the goals of confidentiality outweigh the gains from disclosing information. To use the HIV example above, whether Williams' HIV status should have been disclosed depends on a balance between the general benefits of confidentiality plus Williams' interest in maintaining reputation or in avoiding discrimination, versus the interests of other individuals in avoiding exposure to a chronic and fatal disease. The physician is caught between a duty to the patient versus a duty to the general public (see more complete discussion below).

EXCEPTIONS TO CONFIDENTIALITY

Both the legal and ethical theories reduce to a balance between the interests promoted by confidentiality versus the interests promoted by disclosure. As a result, exceptions should apply when the balance favours disclosure. The following section outlines the mandatory reporting statutes—those that require disclosure to appropriate authorities, as well as the permissive exception statutes—those that allow a physician to use her discretion in deciding whether to disclose information. In the latter situation the statute in question usually provides protections against liability for disclosure. In the former situation, liability may be imposed for failing to disclose. The statutes and case law generally fall into one of four categories: (1) public health, (2) public safety, (3) protection of vulnerable persons, and (4) statistical registries. Each will be addressed in turn.

PUBLIC HEALTH

Physicians have an ethical responsibility to society as well as to individual patients (AMA Opinion 9.07, 1990). This is generally interpreted to mean that physicians have a duty to protect the public health. The extent of this duty is not fully defined, at least with respect to the circumstances under which it outweighs the physician's responsibility to the individual patient. However, there are some clearly articulated limits. For example, a physician cannot experiment on a patient in hopes of benefiting society without the patient's consent when the experiment offers no therapeutic benefit to the patient. In such a case, the obligation to the patient outweighs the obligation to society. But this example refers to a positive duty on the part of the physician—to promote public health. It is less clear how to deal with a negative duty—to prevent harm to the public. May a physician breach confidentiality when public health is threatened?

The most common examples where public health concerns outweigh individual rights of confidentiality are the contagious disease cases (Simonsen v. Swenson, 1920). Most of these cases will not involve neurologists, but some contagious diseases do have neurological implications. Reporting statutes that focus on public health concerns usually mandate disclosure to appropriate public health agencies. But these statutes may also include provisions allowing for disclosure to specific at-risk individuals. A number of states have statutes requiring disclosure of specific diseases such as sexually transmitted diseases (STDs), HIV/AIDS, or general communicable diseases such as tuberculosis (Alabama and Arkansas) and syphilis. Massachusetts requires reporting of Reye's syndrome (M.G.L.A. 111 §110B, 1997), Nevada of epilepsy (N.R.S. §439.270, 1995), and South Carolina of dangerous results from a pathological or bacteriological laboratory. Disclosure may be to public health authorities, other medical care providers (Davis v. Rodman, 1921), partners, family (Skillings v. Allen, 1919), or even needle sharers.

While there have long been reporting statutes for communicable diseases, more recently there has been discussion of a physician's duty to disclose genetic information (Suter, 1994). At least one court has held that a physician may have a duty to disclose genetic information to immediate family members (Safer v. Estate of Pack, 1996). Although genetic traits may be passed on to offspring, they clearly are not transmissible in the same way as contagious diseases and thus should not properly be categorized under public health concerns. The issue of the use of genetic information is beyond the scope of this chapter. Suffice it to say that despite the fact that genetic information may be useful to third parties, this is true of many other types of medical information and should be afforded the same confidentiality protections (Suter, 1994).

Because of the high risk of discrimination and the widespread perception of 'AIDS hysteria', a number of states have passed specific confidentiality legislation for HIV/AIDS. At the same time, numerous states maintain confidential statewide registries in order to keep track of the spread of the virus. For example, New York has strict confidentiality requirements regarding the medical records of HIV/AIDS patients. However, in the light of the Williams case described above there has been a movement to repeal the statute and treat HIV/AIDS like any other communicable disease. This may include mandatory implementation of public health mechanisms such as contact tracing and partner notification (Altman, 1997). Presently, in New York State, individual physicians may conduct partner notifications either in conjunction with, or separately from, public health authorities. However, such mechanisms are used on a voluntary basis and partner notification is generally done without revealing the name of the infected individual. Furthermore, very few individual physicians attempt to implement the notification system. If HIV is treated like other communicable diseases, physicians may have a duty to warn third parties of past or future exposure (Piorkowski, 1987). Duty to warn is discussed in more detail below.

PUBLIC SAFETY

In addition to concerns about public health, there are also a number of situations in which physicians must disclose information in order to safeguard public safety. It is less clear whether physicians have the same ethical responsibility to protect public safety as they do public health. As a result, mandatory reporting statutes in this context may be more problematic from an ethical standpoint. On the other hand, because 'health' is such an expansive concept, it often is difficult to distinguish between concerns about public health and public safety. Many states have reporting statutes for injuries from criminal behaviour, injuries from alcohol, motor vehicle impairments, and burns. Ohio, for example, has a statute mandating the reporting of drug abuse when the individual in question is a public transportation employee (Ohio St. §2305.233, 1997).

Disclosure in these cases usually is to law enforcement authorities. In some cases, however, the physician might be obligated to disclose information to a particular individual or group of individuals. The classic case is the psychotherapist's duty to warn. The concept of a duty to warn in this context originated in a California case, Tarasoff v. Regents of California (1976). In this case, a patient informed his therapist of his intention to kill a young woman. After her death the family sued, claiming that the physician should have warned not only the police but also the victim. The court held that a therapist might be required to reveal information gathered during counselling if the patient's statements indicate that he is likely to seriously injure an identifiable third party. Many states have adopted this doctrine and some have extended it to all physicians or mental health professionals. Duty to warn cases focus on (1) the seriousness of the threat of harm, and (2) the identifiability of the victim. Thus a physician is not under an obligation to reveal threats of minor harm, threats that the physician does not believe are serious, or general threats where there is no identifiable third party.

> Mr A is a 45-year-old school bus driver who has been referred to Dr Smith for repeated 'blackouts'. Dr Smith diagnoses epilepsy and prescribes Dilantin. Mr A is concerned that he will lose his job if his employer finds out about his medical condition. Dr Smith has an obligation to warn Mr A about the potential risks of his driving. In addition, since Mr A is a school bus driver, Dr Smith has an obligation to report his seizures to the appropriate authorities, thus preventing him from driving until his disorder is under control.

PROTECTION OF VULNERABLE PERSONS

Less controversial than the public safety cases are the protection of vulnerable persons cases. Although physicians have at least some responsibility to safeguard vulnerable persons (e.g., sick patients), it is not clear whether this duty extends to the general public, nor whether it should outweigh individual confidentiality protections. With respect to minors, however, these protections are generally thought to be appropriate. Almost all states have child abuse reporting statutes. Missouri specifically requires physicians to report drug-dependent minors to the health department (Mo. St. §191.737, 1997). New Jersey expands the requirement to all drug-dependent patients (N.J.S.A. §24:21–39, 1997). In addition, some states have statutes that require reporting of abuse of hospital patients or long-term care patients, elder abuse, spousal abuse, and domestic abuse.

Reporting of drug abuse, spousal abuse and domestic abuse are more controversial than child or elder abuse. Children and elderly persons are particularly vulnerable to abuse. It is not as clear whether the balance works in favour of disclosure for drug abuse or spousal/domestic abuse. There is a high likelihood that these individuals may not seek needed help and treatment if they fear disclosure. Some commentators argue that where the abused individual is a competent adult and would prefer to keep the information confidential, his or her wishes should be respected. The AMA *Code of Medical Ethics*, for example, stresses that abuse involving competent adults should not be disclosed without consent (Opinion 2.02). On the other hand, without mandatory reporting requirements, individuals may be trapped indefinitely in abusive relationships.[6]

> The school nurse refers T to a primary care physician for a medical evaluation after she complains of severe headaches and difficulty concentrating in classes. The primary care physician refers T to Dr Jones, a neurologist, for evaluation of the headaches. During the course of evaluation, Dr Jones suspects focal seizures probably originating from trauma to the girl's skull. He suspects that T's problems might arise from child abuse. Dr Jones has an obligation to report the suspected abuse to the appropriate authorities.

STATISTICAL REGISTRIES

Finally, sometimes disclosure is required for informational purposes. Disclosure in these cases is usually the least controversial since the information is provided to state or federal agencies and not disclosed to the public. The data gathered is incorporated into registries that allow officials to keep various statistics. These may be found in conjunction with public health reporting requirements, e.g. HIV/AIDS registries; another example is cancer registries. In addition, Kansas keeps track of children with developmental disabilities, and Maine requires reporting of occupational diseases. These registries are usually kept confidential, and in some cases data may be maintained without identifiers.

Recently however, there have been a number of concerns raised about such databases, especially when the information stored can be linked to identifiers, or is stored in computer banks (Woodward, 1997). Genetic or other sensitive information databases raise additional concerns, particularly if law enforcement officials may access the information (Turkington, 1997). Attention in this area is presently focused less on state registries per se, and more on the need to develop better security mechanisms in order to ensure the continued confidentiality of medical information in the age of computerization and telemedicine (Rind *et al.*, 1997; Sweeny, 1997).

> Dr Snow has recently been notified that the state in which she lives is collecting information about multiple sclerosis. She has a number of MS patients. The state requires listings of all patients with MS, including sex and age of onset of symptoms. It does not, however, require

[6]There is little evidence one way or the other about the benefits of reporting in this context.

inclusion of patient names or other identifying information. Dr Snow should comply with the requirement.

DISCLOSURE IN OTHER CIRCUMSTANCES

Besides the general issue of confidentiality within the traditional patient–physician relationship, there are a few other situations that are relevant. Physicians who perform examinations for insurance companies or employers (AMA, Opinion 5.09, 1996), or who take part in court-ordered evaluations will often be required to disclose their findings even without the patient's consent. Technically one might argue that there is no patient–physician relationship in these cases, and thus no duty to maintain confidentiality. However, because patients may not be aware of the intricacies of this type of encounter, physicians should make the limits of confidentiality clear from the outset using principles of informed consent. Thus these situations are best looked at not as exceptions to confidentiality, but as cases where the scope of the physician's duty to disclose information to a third party is established as part of the initial agreement between the patient and physician.

> Mr C is a 55-year-old defendant in a vehicular homicide case who is referred to Dr Smith, a neurologist, by the court to evaluate his claim that he had a seizure that caused him to lose control of his automobile. During the course of the interview Dr Smith finds no structural cause for the seizure, but does believe that the evidence points to a high likelihood of substance abuse. Dr Smith is required to include this information in his report to the court.

CONCLUSION

Confidentiality in medical practice is a strong requirement but is not absolute. Physicians need to be aware of the multitude of exceptions to confidentiality. While this need not entail memorization of the different reporting laws, it should involve an understanding of the ethical basis for confidentiality protections as well as a familiarity with the general categories of exceptions. Neurologists, like other physicians, may be required to disclose information when there is a threat to the public health or safety (e.g. dangerous drivers), a need to protect vulnerable persons such as children or the elderly, or to statistical registries for diseases such as Creutzfeldt–Jakob or amyotrophic lateral sclerosis (ALS).

REFERENCES

Altman (1997) Sex, privacy and tracking HIV infections. *New York Times* November 4.
American Medical Association (1990) *Code of Medical Ethics.*
American Medical Association (1996) *Principles of Medical Ethics, Preamble.*

Cruzan v. Director, Missouri Dept of Health, 497 U.W. 261, 1990.

Davis H (1997) Latest tests reveal Williams allegedly infected 13 women. *The Buffalo News* December 10, 4B.

Davis v. Rodman, 227 S.W. 612, 1921.

Frankel T (1983) Fiduciary law. *California Law Review* **71**:795–836.

Friedland B (1994) Patient-physician confidentiality, *Journal of Legal Medicine* **15**:249–277, 256–57.

Gellman R (1984) Prescribing privacy: The uncertain role of the physician in the protection of patient privacy. *North Carolina Law Review* **62**:255–294, 267.

Horne v. Patton, 287 So.2d 824, Ala. 1973.

McConnell T (1994) Confidentiality and the law. *Journal of Medical Ethics* **20**:47–49.

Murphy R (1996) Property rights in personal information: An economic defense of privacy. *Georgetown Law Journal* **84**:2381–2417.

Piorkowski J (1987) Between a rock and a hard place: AIDS and the conflicting physician's duties of preventing disease transmission and safeguarding confidentiality. *Georgetown Law Journal* **76**:169–202.

Restatement Second of Agency 395, 1958.

Rind D, Kohane I, Szolovits P *et al.* (1997) Maintaining confidentiality of medical records shared over the internet and the world wide web. *Annals of Internal Medicine* **127**:138–141.

Rodwin M (1995) Strains in the fiduciary metaphor: Divided physician loyalties and obligation in a changing health care system. *American Journal of Law & Medicine* **21**:241–257.

Safer v. Estate of Pack, 677 A.2d 1188, 1996.

Scalen E (1991) Promises broken v. promises betrayed: Metaphor, analogy, and the new fiduciary principle. *University of Illinois Law Review*: 897–980.

Simonsen v. Swenson, 177 N.W. 831, 1920.

Skillings v. Allen, 173 N.W. 663, 1919.

Smith S (1986) Medical and psychotherapy privileges and confidentiality: On giving with one hand and removing with the other. *Kentucky Law Journal* **75**:473–557.

Stein M, Freedberg K, Sullivan L *et al.* (1998) Sexual ethics: Disclosure of HIV-positive status to partners. *Archives of Internal Medicine* **158**:253–257.

Suter S (1994) Whose genes are these anyway? Familial conflicts over access to genetic information. *Michigan Law Review* **91**:1854–1908.

Sweeny L (1997) Weaving technology and policy together to maintain confidentiality. *Journal of Law, Medicine & Ethics* **25**:98–110.

Tarasoff v. Regents of California, 551 P.2d 334, Cal. 1976.

Temkin O and Temkin C, eds (1967) *Ancient Medicine: Selected Papers of Ludwig Edelstein*. Baltimore: Johns Hopkins University Press.

Turkington R (1997) Medical record confidentiality: Law, scientific research, and data collection in the information age. *Journal of Law, Medicine & Ethics* **25**:113–129.

United States Const. Amend. IV.

United States Dept of Justice v. Reporters' Comm. 489 U.W. 749, 763, 1989.

Woodward B (1997) Medical record confidentiality and data collection: Current dilemmas. *Journal of Law, Medicine & Ethics* **25**:88–97.

Therapy

7

Why, and How, Should Trials Be Conducted?

Richard I Lindley, Charles P Warlow

ABSTRACT

In this essay we argue that doctors have an ethical imperative to participate in randomized controlled trials (RCTs) as part of their duty to improve the care they offer their patients. Many of the ethical dilemmas associated with RCTs are actually due to poor methodology and bad science. Good trial design and sound science with peer review can eliminate these. We emphasize the importance of true randomization (to avoid any systematic bias) and large studies (to avoid random error and so reduce the chance of false negative and false positive results). Consent is puzzling to many doctors and patients and we illustrate 'how to do it' with examples from our own busy clinical practice. Consent is all about giving patients enough information to enable them to decide whether or not they take part in a RCT. Like all consultations, this requires an individualized approach adapted to that particular patient's circumstances. Neurological disease can often render patients mentally incompetent and we explain how it is still ethical to randomize these patients. There is no doubt that doctors and our patients need far more education about RCTs, and we need to discuss difficult ethical issues with our local population, doctors and ethicists.

INTRODUCTION

In this essay we outline why clinical trials are an essential part of modern neurological practice and compare them with routine clinical practice. We then discuss how to do clinical trials and point out areas that some find ethically difficult. We will not hide our enthusiasm for randomized controlled trials and we hope that this chapter will explode a few myths and challenge the view that clinical trials are an ethical minefield.

THE IMPERATIVE TO PERFORM CLINICAL TRIALS

Doctors have an ethical imperative to identify advances in health care (Cancer Research Campaign Working Party in Breast Conservation, 1983; American Medical Association, 1996). The enormous advances in health in the twentieth century have arisen for two main reasons: better environmental conditions (e.g. safe water) and advances in health care (e.g. near eradication of polio by vaccination). But no-one argues that we have now reached the end of medical progress, and if doctors are to improve the health of their patients further, they need to constantly improve their practice. We will clearly maximize our achievements if we all contribute to this progress. After all, if we do not do the research, no-one else is going to do it for us. Careful observation and description were the cornerstones of previous medical progress but we now have far more sophisticated and reliable methods for demonstrating advances in health care. It is interesting to note that many of the recent advances in neurology have involved very large collaborative groups including some doctors who may not have done much research in the past (e.g. the European Atrial Fibrillation Trial Collaborative Group). Doctors need to identify effective treatments and discard treatments which prove to be harmful. The most cost-effective and reliable way to do this is by the RCT.

Why is the RCT the most effective way of evaluating a treatment strategy? Despite much wishful thinking there are really no alternatives, and it is useful to explore the reasons for this. In neurology, like most of medicine, major treatment effects are rare (try and think of some). Most treatments only offer a modest (or moderate) benefit which is difficult to identify unless great care is taken to eliminate or reduce moderate biases in their evaluation (Yusuf *et al.*, 1984).

The assessment of treatment effects would be easy if we were able accurately to predict every patient's outcome for every disease. Clinical experience tells us that this is completely unrealistic. *Exactly* when will Mrs X, who has motor neurone disease, die? *Precisely* when will the disabled stroke patient start walking without a walking stick? On what day *exactly* will the next relapse of multiple sclerosis occur? We simply do not know the answers to these rather simple questions, yet our patients are often surprised by this sort of ignorance. Patients differ so much from each other that we can only estimate prognosis with and without treatment by studying large groups of people. The main purpose of randomization is to establish two (or more) groups of patients that are as similar as possible in all known, and even unknown, ways. So, after the treatment is applied to one group and not the other, and the two groups differ by a statistically significant amount in some outcome measure (e.g. death or dependency), we can assume that this difference must be the sole result of the treatment. This can be compared with the common clinical practice of only using the interesting, fashionable or favoured treatments on patients who were going to do well anyway. Sackett (1989) has summarized the results of such practice with the comment: 'Therapeutic reports with controls tend to have no enthusiasm, and reports with enthusiasm tend to have no controls'. Only randomization can reliably eliminate a systematic bias in the comparison of treated and untreated groups of subjects in a clinical trial.

TRUE RANDOMIZATION

The essential features of secure randomization in a clinical trial are:

The randomizing person must not be able to predict the treatment allocation in advance. Methods such as the use of the hospital number, date of birth or alternate allocation are inadequate. Although some of these, at face value, may look reasonable, they all permit subversion of the randomization process and the introduction of bias (consciously or subconsciously) by allowing the doctor to give the test treatment to patients who may well have a good outcome even if untreated. Such methods have certainly produced substantial bias in previous trials (Wright *et al.*, 1948).

Once randomized, the patient cannot be withdrawn from the study (otherwise faultless randomization, such as by sealed envelope, can sometimes be subverted in this way). Bias can occur if, for example, a treatment makes some patients who are destined to do badly feel unwell and stop the treatment, not get followed up, and so not be analysed; the treatment group will then have, on average, a better outcome than would in fact have been the case if all patients had been followed up and analysed. The 'intention-to-treat' analysis avoids this sort of bias.

The randomization method should be designed to create two groups of subjects who are as similar as possible to each other. This is usually done by generating treatment allocation by a random method, now most often done by computer. Some methods of randomization manipulate the allocation to balance the treatment groups by important prognostic baseline data, such as the minimization method (White and Freedman, 1993). Strictly speaking, minimization is not actually random but in practice it achieves the required end result (two groups that are as similar as possible in their prognosis at baseline).

LARGE SAMPLE SIZE, THE ELIMINATION OF CHANCE EFFECTS

It follows from the above argument that if we, as doctors, are unable to predict clinical outcome accurately, chance effects may well influence the outcomes seen in some groups of patients. Thus, the other main source of error in clinical trials is the play of chance leading to imprecision of the trial result (i.e. false positive or negative results). Random error is often far more powerful than the treatment effect under study and most clinical trials in neurology have been hopelessly underpowered to detect the sort of modest treatment effects that are common in medicine. Part of this is due to the unrealistic optimism of the research neurologist, but a general ignorance of unavoidable statistical imperatives has also played a major part.

In summary, a secure method of randomization to eliminate systematic bias and large numbers of subjects to reduce random error are the key ingredients of a good trial.

RANDOMIZED CONTROLLED TRIALS VERSUS CLINICAL PRACTICE

Randomized controlled trials differ from routine clinical practice in the following ways:

(1) The treatment (or management protocol) is likely to have been thoroughly peer reviewed by colleagues, grant-giving bodies and ethics committees. On the other hand, in normal clinical practice, treatment can be given on the say so of just one possibly ignorant, biased or corrupt doctor.

(2) There are detailed clinical records which are usually kept for years, long after many hospital or office records are destroyed.

(3) Diagnosis and treatment are likely to be performed systematically according to a research protocol. In normal clinical practice there are still few guidelines that are adhered to.

(4) Patients are carefully monitored and great efforts are made to provide a systematic and complete follow-up—quite unlike normal clinical practice where patients can easily be lost to follow-up or deliberately discharged.

(5) The responsible clinicians are often national (or local) experts and so the trial has an educational role for less expert collaborators.

(6) The management is audited and treatment success or failure is monitored, with the responsible clinicians informed of significant risks or benefits as soon as they are discovered by the data monitoring committee.

(7) Treatment allocation is determined by randomization.

It is therefore no surprise that patients in RCTs tend to do better than those in routine clinical practice (Stiller, 1994; Hancock *et al.*, 1997). Furthermore, it seems perverse that so much fuss is made about the last point (random allocation of treatment) and that all the others are so often completely ignored. Before we discuss the whole issue of randomization it is worth pointing out that points 1–6 hide a few important ethical issues.

A good clinical trial should be based on good medical science, and peer review is a key to this. Bad or shoddy designs should be eliminated early. To protect the patients, all trials, even those which do not need external funding, should be reviewed by an ethics committee. If an institution does not have an ethics committee (or equivalent) it must be a priority to create one (Royal College of Physicians, 1990a). The trial should be monitored in some way. This may take the form of a named clinician in each centre taking responsibility for data collection and ensuring good quality care in the trial. Good management should also include an audit of data (data checking) and ideally an audit of the actual documentation (site visits, etc.) to ensure that all is well.

A key ethical part of the trial design is external data monitoring and occasional interim analyses. Data should be observed by an independent statistician who can notify the trial organizers (such as a steering committee) if one treatment is significantly beneficial or hazardous. These sorts of data should be presented in an anonymized way to the steering committee for them to make a judgement that the trial should be stopped or allowed to continue.

If an RCT satisfies points 1–6 above, many of the arguments about randomization and consent disappear. In our opinion, most of the arguments about the ethics of randomization have really been misdirected arguments about trial design (points 1–6) and are, in a sense, beside the point.

ETHICAL ISSUES

In our opinion, clinical trial medicine differs from routine clinical practice in two ethical requirements:

(1) The patients give consent to be the subject in a research project, whether or not it involves randomization, because they are then allowing themselves, in some sense, to be 'experimented on' and their possibly very private details to be used for research.
(2) The patients and responsible clinicians must be happy that the treatment allocation is by a random method; in other words that an individual patient does not definitely need one of the treatments under evaluation (or definitely not need it).

The second point clearly does not apply to research projects that do not include randomization such as cohort studies or other forms of observational epidemiology. The point we particularly wish to emphasize is that clinical standards should be similar in research and routine clinical practice. We must avoid double standards.

CONSENT

In our view 'consent' (or 'informed consent') means that the patients understand they are to be in a research project with the aim of identifying what treatment (or management strategy) is best for patients like themselves (Royal College of Physicians, 1990b). Patients need to be told, according to their individual wishes and understanding, the known risks and possible benefits of the different treatments under evaluation and should be given an opportunity to ask pertinent questions and have time for reflection (Cancer Research Campaign Working Party in Breast Conservation, 1983). This process is often helped by providing written material which should be simple to read (e.g. language understandable by grade 5 or 11 year olds), informative, and contain details of the responsible clinician and institution (address and telephone number, etc.). Those with word processors can check the readability of their prose by the automated grammar check software.

Consent should definitely not involve a long document detailing every single imaginable potential risk and benefit of all the treatments in enormous detail, anymore than in routine clinical practice. Such documents are clearly not protecting the patient but protecting the doctor, and they can become a prohibitive barrier to reasonable participation (Taylor *et al.*, 1984). A detailed account of the consent procedure for the landmark ISIS-2 trial in the US has been published by Collins *et al.* (1992). They calculated that the consent procedure probably caused the premature death of 10 000 patients world-wide as a result of poor recruitment rates in the US which led to a delay in completing the trial. Ethicists who demand protracted consent procedures should be aware of the risks of such 'delaying' behaviour.

Obtaining consent is an individualized procedure involving a core of information supplemented by additional material as deemed appropriate by the randomizing clinician (Wager *et al.*, 1995). For example in a recent trial that we were involved with, we randomized patients with acute ischaemic stroke to one of six combinations of aspirin, heparin or no antithrombitic (International Stroke Trial Collaborative Group, 1997). Some consent procedures were very brief, others were protracted and involved many parties. The key element of a successful consent procedure is judging the amount of information to be imparted, being humane and assessing understanding. A five-minute discussion with verbal consent was often appropriate when talking to an older frightened patient with a left hemiparesis.

Are there situations where consent need not be obtained?

This is a controversial area and there is no easy answer. A recent trial from our unit was done without informed consent, with our local ethics committee's agreement (Dennis *et al.*, 1997). We were evaluating a family support worker whose role was to support patients (and their carers) after a hospital admission for acute stroke. We only obtained consent for a detailed follow-up after hospital discharge. We were concerned that a consent procedure for the randomized trial part of the project might have biased the trial by making the control group feel neglected (Dennis, 1997). As we were measuring many aspects of outcome, including psychological well-being, there was a real problem of dangling an apparently attractive option (a support worker) in front of the patient and then denying half the patients that option. The trial result surprised us. The group of patients allocated support by the worker appeared to become more helpless, less well adjusted and more depressed than the control group. The lack of consent was criticized by ethicists who argued that the loss of patient autonomy (i.e. not knowing the full facts of the research project) was not worth the control of bias in the trial design (McLean, 1997). Another lesson from this project is that there may be unexpected adverse effects that none of the researchers expect, and you simply cannot assume that an unproven treatment (or other intervention) is really entirely without risk.

Consent procedures for patients who are dysphasic or unconscious

Under English law no-one can give consent apart from the patient, but this has not stopped trials including patients who are unable to give consent (e.g. the International Stroke Trial). Most ethics committees in the United Kingdom have pragmatically accepted that assent by relatives (or even by independent persons) is a valid method of protecting patients. If dysphasic patients were always excluded from randomized trials, they, as a group, would never benefit from better treatment because we would never be able to reliably evaluate them, an unacceptable ethical position.

Patients who are unconscious are often treated by doctors in routine clinical practice without consent from anyone, let alone the patient. Our ethical duty (under common law) to provide care overwhelms the lack of consent in this emergency situation. If a doctor believes there are two possible treatments which are applicable in this emergency situation he can give either treatment without fear of being accused of unlawful behaviour. Paradoxically, if the same doctor were to give one of the treatments as a result of random allocation in a well-designed clinical trial to find out which one worked best, he could be tried in a court of law for battery (although this has never been tested in the UK). This double standard has been recognized for some time and Institutional Review Boards in the USA allow randomization into RCTs provided strict criteria are followed:

(1) The patient's relatives are unavailable or the trial treatment must be administered before consent from the legally authorized representatives is feasible.
(2) The patient has a life-threatening condition with only unproven treatments available.
(3) The patient is unable to give consent because of his or her medical condition.

Consent for those who are incompetent

Some have suggested that randomization without consent is ethically acceptable for the mentally incompetent, provided the risks are not too great (Doyal, 1997), but others have argued that this is too restrictive and will condemn many patients with severe illness, when a risky treatment might be worthwhile, to no prospect of better care (Lindley, 1998).

Ethically, doctors have a duty to improve the care of patients who, by reason of accident or pathology are mentally incompetent (e.g. following head injury). It is therefore illogical to refuse to consider such patients for RCTs merely because they are unable to give consent. Provided suitable safeguards are present we see no barrier to such patients being included in RCTs. The necessary safeguards must include good science (see above) and all projects should be scrutinized by local ethics committees. In this particular area we believe the public should be part of the discussion. If lay people contribute to and inform the trial consent procedure there is less likelihood of abuse of patients in research protocols. One idea suggested has been the introduction of a 'randomized controlled trial' card. This card would give an advance directive (in a similar way to kidney donor cards) to any RCT which has proper ethics committee approval in the event of the card holder suddenly becoming mentally incompetent but eligible for an appropriate RCT (Lindley, 1998). If such a card were established it might increase public knowledge of RCTs and stimulate discussion on their merits and the ethical dilemmas that arise.

'Not in my backyard'

The 'not-in-my-backyard' or NIMBY mentality, is as prominent in medicine as in contemporary politics. People want the best treatment for themselves but perhaps not what they see as the personal risks involved in taking part in an RCT. Ethically, should the middle class populace demand the best treatments (identified by RCTs) and at the same time refuse consent into RCTs that may be offered to them? (Baum, 1995). Should the battle of disease control be fought only by those who meekly accept randomization offered by the enthusiastic trialist? Some have compared this to wars being fought only by the dispossessed youth of society (Baum, personal communication). Another double standard is practised by health purchasers who demand evidence based medicine but do not invest in public health and educational campaigns to increase public knowledge of RCTs. Perhaps the RCT card will help in this matter. The public ought to be informed about the burning questions in medicine and the need for clinical trials which will help resolve uncertainties. There is some evidence that this can improve recruitment, and lay contribution to clinical trials will benefit us all (Thornton, 1993; Chalmers, 1995).

Alternatives to traditional consent

Some have suggested an alternative method of randomization which aims to maintain the scientific advantages of true randomization but makes consent procedures easier. This is illustrated in Fig. 7.1 (Zelen, 1990). Essentially, eligible patients are randomized before the consent consultation. There is therefore an element of certainty in the discussion as the researcher can ask permission for trial entry and discuss the pros and cons of the (randomly) allocated treatment.

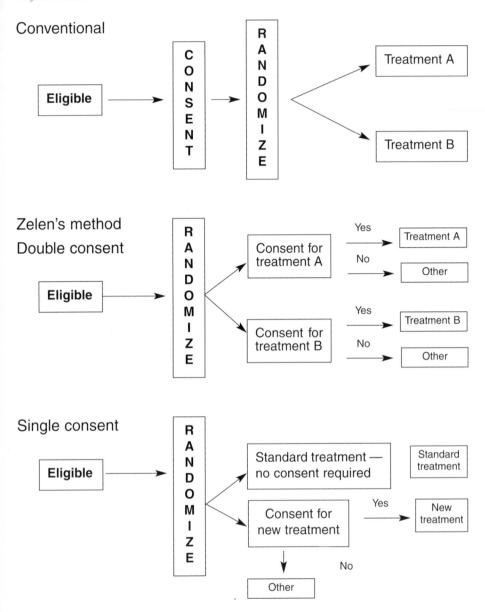

Figure 7.1 Flow diagrams illustrating a conventional randomization and consent procedure and Zelen's alternatives.

This method may be acceptable provided that there is not a large refusal rate, which would damage the study, especially if the refusal rates were significantly different between the treatment groups. A slight modification of this method of randomization was successfully used in a recent trial of a policy of discharging patients home early (with intensive community support and rehabilitation) after a hospital admission for stroke (Rodgers *et al.*, 1997). All patients were approached for consent to data collection. Those randomized to routine hospital care were not approached again, but merely followed up because this was normal practice. Those allocated the new policy of early supported discharge were re-interviewed and consent was obtained for the new policy. In the Newcastle trial, few refused consent at this second stage.

Written or verbal consent?

There should be no legal or ethical difference between these two methods, although written consent has the advantage of providing a permanent record. But written consent can have disadvantages, especially for older people. We have had experience of this a few years ago when one of us was obtaining consent from an older patient for entry into a secondary prevention trial (the CAPRIE trial). The patient listened carefully to all the arguments, including the statement that she was free to leave the study at any time without penalty. However, when presented with the written consent form she commented that this 'must be legally binding' if she had to sign it. Written consent can so easily allow the patient to believe that he or she has 'signed my rights away'. One way around this problem is to state to the potential subject 'I would like you to sign this form which summarizes our discussion and provides proof that I (the doctor) have done my job properly'. By switching the emphasis on to the doctor many patients feel less threatened.

THE 'UNCERTAINTY PRINCIPLE'

We believe this principle has been a very important advance in the ethics of the RCT. The guiding principle is that doctors should always use treatments and management strategies if they are certain they are effective. Similarly, no doctor should use a treatment which he or she is certain is ineffective. However, if the doctor, in consultation with a patient, is uncertain of the best treatment strategy, given more than one option, the best resolution of this uncertainty is randomization in a well-designed RCT. The advantages of this principle are many: all patients get treatments their doctor is certain about; no patient receives treatment the doctor believes to be ineffective; and with RCTs we all learn something useful. Where uncertainty lies, an answer will emerge from the RCT. The patient–doctor relationship is preserved if the uncertainty principle is followed and therefore doctors can adhere to the time honoured Hippocratic ethos of always doing the best for the patient in front of them.

We believe another advantage to be that the 'uncertainty principle' defines what is scientifically interesting and encourages doctors to explore new treatments with the knowledge that their patients are furthering medical knowledge. To illustrate this principle we reproduce our guide to randomizing a patient into the International Stroke Trial that evaluated immediate aspirin and heparin for acute ischaemic stroke (Fig. 7.2).

Ethics and the International Stroke Trial (IST)

Suggestions on how clinicians might discuss entry in the IST with patients who have been admitted to hospital with an acute stroke

A fundamental principle of the IST is that eligibility is governed by the uncertainty principle:

Patients are eligible for IST if the doctor is substantially **uncertain** of the benefit of IST treatments **for that particular patient.**

Patients are **not** eligible if the doctor is reasonably **certain** that any one of the IST treatments is clearly indicated or contraindicated.

Consent procedure

This is a matter for individual doctors to decide for individual patients and needs to take into account local regulations and advice from local ethical committees. But above all, must be humane for patients at an obviously distressing time. Prolonged consent procedures with a compulsory written consent should be avoided as this can sometimes **cause** unnecessary distress and would, in this situation, be unethical.

Structure of suggested informed consent procedure

Discuss the potential benefits

After discussing the likely diagnosis with the patient, you can explain:

"For patients with **your** particular type of stroke there is no treatment that has clearly been shown to be effective. The stroke has most likely been caused by a blood clot blocking an artery, and 'blood thinning' treatments like aspirin and heparin may be beneficial. Treatment may improve the chance of making a good recovery (and prevent blood clots forming in the leg veins) and we know that these treatments work for other similar medical problems that are also due to blood clots (e.g. heart attacks)."

Explain the potential risks of treatments

"Like all 'blood thinning' treatments, aspirin and heparin can cause bleeding, although the risk of a serious bleed is small. The heparin injections often cause trivial colouration at the site of injection and occasionally can be uncomfortable. Aspirin can cause stomach irritation but allergic reactions are very rare.

We are doing this study in order to find out the best treatment for patients like yourself, and to make sure that there are no important side effects. For you, the best option is not clear:
a) Should we give the 'blood thinning' treatment aspirin immediately, or
b) Should we wait for a couple of weeks, to reduce the risk of side effects?

And similarly:
a) Should we give you heparin, another 'blood thinning' treatment immediately, or
b) Would it be better to avoid it for at least two weeks, because it might cause side-effects?

Would you be happy to take part in this study?

If **yes**, we will use one of several combinations of aspirin and heparin (or avoid using them) for a few weeks (or until you're well enough to go home). The aspirin is given as one tablet a day (or a suppository if you cannot swallow). The heparin is given as small injections twice daily into your skin (this sometimes causes some discolouration). There are no extra tests or clinic visits, we simply contact you in about six months (by post or telephone) to find out how you are getting on.

If I, or any other doctor looking after you, believe it necessary to change your treatment or withdraw you from the study, we will. You will, at all times, get any treatment we think will definitely help. Whether or not you decide to join the study you will get the best management we can provide. If you do decide to join, you are free to withdraw from the study at any time.

To find out what treatment you will get, I will phone the study co-ordinators who are based in Oxford. Your details will be fed into a computer and a specific treatment will be allocated for you."

Record any consent obtained in the hospital records

If appropriate, give the patient and/or relatives the IST information leaflet.

Make phone call to Oxford, record the allocation in the patients' notes and write up any active treatment to be given immediately.

Tell the patient and/or relatives what you are going to use.

Figure 7.2 This training document was used for the United Kingdom International Stroke Trial Collaborators. This study was a very large 'mega-trial' testing immediate aspirin, subcutaneous heparin (in two doses), both or neither for patients with ischaemic stroke. We found it very useful to help guide junior doctors in the sort of consent consultation we found useful and non-threatening, based on our experience in the pilot study (International Stroke Trial Collaborative Group, 1997).

The advantages of the 'uncertainty principle' were also seen in the European Carotid Surgery Trial (European Carotid Surgery Trialists' Collaborative Group, 1998). Neurologists and surgeons were asked to randomize patients with a recent symptomatic carotid territory ischaemic event for whom they were uncertain about having a carotid endarterectomy in addition to 'best medical care'. Some were only uncertain about the value of carotid endarterectomy if the stenosis was very severe; these doctors therefore only randomized patients with severe stenosis. Others only randomized those with mild stenosis as they were certain that patients with high-grade stenosis should be operated on. Some were uncertain about the value of the operation in any patient and therefore randomized all grades of stenosis. Overall, many hundreds of patients with mild, moderate and severe stenosis were randomized, providing a uniquely useful database of the value of carotid surgery for stenosis ranging from 0 to 99%. A North American study did not use the uncertainty principle; patients with mild carotid stenosis were not eligible, and so this study was not able to show that the net effect of surgery was harmful for them (North American Symptomatic Carotid Endarterectomy Trial Collaborative Group, 1991). The evidence that carotid surgery was not beneficial for those with mild stenosis came mainly from the European study which, by using the 'uncertainty principle', had more flexible eligibility criteria and thus was able to answer more questions than the North American trial.

We believe that more widespread use of the uncertainty principle will encourage greater recruitment into RCTs and allow greater clinical freedom. This will provide a broader range of patients in RCTs, which should increase the generalizability of the trial results (by being less restrictive) and the scientific interest of the study.

TRAINING ISSUES

The concept, rationale and design of RCTs needs to be an early component of training of young doctors (and other health professionals), and courses should be available to teach others 'how to do it'. We believe that RCTs should be part of our routine clinical practice. We use treatments we believe to be effective, we avoid those we believe to be useless (or harmful), and we randomize patients between treatments we are uncertain about until that uncertainty is resolved.

FINANCIAL MATTERS AND SCIENTIFIC FRAUD

Sadly, there have been several examples of scientific fraud in RCTs in recent times. There are many reasons why some may be tempted to augment patient recruitment by fraudulent means including: the need to impress their peers; the need for publications to further their careers; and financial inducements that are greater than the costs of recruiting patients.

Our local ethics committee now asks for details of financial rewards in order to scrutinize trials that may be overgenerous and encourage fraud. One recent example of RCT fraud was identified by good central data checking (Diener *et al.*, 1996). Data can be inspected for fraud as it is extremely difficult to fabricate 'random' data; unusual non-random data from individual investigators should prompt an audit of primary data and medical records. Trial data sets can be monitored for such non-random data and this should be part of the internal consistency checks of a major trial.

FINAL CONCLUSIONS

We believe that the key ingredients of an ethical clinical trial are good science, along with honest (but humane) discussion with our patients and their relatives and carers. When dealing with difficult ethical issues, local experts and ethics committees should be consulted. Clinical trials should be part of every neurologist's clinical practice if they are to keep at the cutting edge of their speciality.

REFERENCES

American Medical Association (1996) *Code of Medical Ethics: Current Opinions and Annotations.* (http://www.ama-assn.org/ethic/pome.htm)

Baum M (1995) The ethics of randomized controlled trials. *European Journal of Surgical Oncology* **21**:136–139.

Cancer Research Campaign Working Party in Breast Conservation (1983) Informed consent: ethical, legal, and medical implications for doctors and patients who participate in randomised clinical trials. *British Medical Journal* **286**:1117–1221.

Chalmers I (1995) What do I want from health research and researchers when I am a patient? *British Medical Journal* **310**:1315–1318.

Collins R, Doll R and Peto R (1992) Ethics of clinical trials. In: *Introducing New Treatments for Cancer: Practical, Ethical and Legal Problems* (ed CJ Williams), pp. 49–65. Chichester: John Wiley & Sons.

Dennis M (1997) Commentary: Why we didn't ask patients for their consent. *British Medical Journal* **314**:1077.

Dennis M, O'Rourke S, Slattery J, Staniforth T and Warlow C (1997) Evaluation of a stroke family care worker: results of a randomised controlled trial. *British Medical Journal* **314**:1071–1077.

Diener HC, Cunha L, Forbes C, Sivenius J, Smets P and Lowenthal A (1996) European Stroke Prevention Study 2. Dipyridamole and acetylsalicylic acid in the secondary prevention of stroke. *Journal of the Neurological Sciences* **143**:1–13.

Doyal L (1997) Informed consent in medical research. *British Medical Journal* **314**:1107–1111.

European Carotid Surgery Trial Collaborative Group. (1998) Randomised trial of endarterectomy for recently symptomatic carotid stenosis: final results of the MRC European Carotid Surgery Trial (ECST). *Lancet* **351**:1379–1387.

Hancock BW, Aitken M, Radstone C and Vaughan Hudson G (1997) Why don't cancer patients get entered into clinical trials? Experience of the Sheffield Lymphoma Group's collaboration in British National Lymphoma Investigation studies. *British Medical Journal* **314**:36–37.

International Stroke Trial Collaborative Group (1997) The International Stroke Trial (IST): a randomised trial of aspirin, subcutaneous heparin, both, or neither among 19435 patients with acute ischaemic stroke. *Lancet* **349**:1569–1581.

Lindley RI (1998) Thrombolytic treatment for acute ischaemic stroke: consent can be ethical. *British Medical Journal* **316**:1005–1007.

McLean S (1997) Commentary: No consent means not treating the patient with respect. *British Medical Journal* **314**:1076.

North American Symptomatic Carotid Endarterectomy Trial Collaborative Group. (1991) Beneficial effect of carotid endarterectomy in symptomatic patients with high-grade carotid stenosis. *New England Journal of Medicine* **325**:445–453.

Rodgers H, Soutter J, Kaiser W *et al.* (1997) Early supported discharge following acute stroke—a randomised controlled trial: pilot study results. *Clinical Rehabilitation* **11**:280–287.

Royal College of Physicians (1990a) *Guidelines on the Practice of Ethics Committees in Medical Research Involving Human Subjects*, 2nd edn. London: The Royal College of Physicians of London.

Royal College of Physicians (1990b). *Research Involving Patients*. London: The Royal College of Physicians of London.

Sackett DL (1989) Rules of evidence and clinical recommendations on the use of antithrombotic agents. *Chest* **89** (suppl. 2):S2–S3.

Stiller CA (1994) Centralised treatment, entry to trials and survival. *British Journal of Cancer* **70**:352–362.

Taylor KM, Margolese RG and Soskolne CL (1984) Physicians' reasons for not entering eligible patients in a randomized clinical trial of surgery for breast cancer. *New England Journal of Medicine* **310**:1363–1367.

Thornton H (1993) Clinical trials: a 'ladyplan' for trial recruitment?—everyone's business. *Lancet* **341**:795–796.

Wager E, Tooley PJH, Emanuel MB and Wood SF (1995) How to do it? Get patients' consent to enter clinical trials. *British Medical Journal* **311**:734–737.

White SJ and Freedman LS (1993) Allocation of patients to treatment groups in a controlled clinical study. *British Journal of Cancer* **37**:849–857.

Wright IS, Marple CD and Beck DF (1948) Report of the committee for the evaluation of anticoagulants in the treatment of coronary thrombosis with myocardial infarction. *American Heart Journal* **36**:801.

Yusuf S, Collins R and Peto R (1984) Why do we need some large, simple randomised trials? *Statistics in Medicine* **3**:409–420.

Zelen M (1990) Randomized consent designs for clinical trials: an update. *Statistics in Medicine* **9**:645–656.

8

How Should We Test and Improve Neurosurgical Care?

Grant Gillett

ABSTRACT

The introduction of new surgical techniques is problematic and requires that special account be taken of the evolving and practical nature of surgery. The fact that surgeons are practising a craft entails a constant search for ways to improve their skills. Sometimes these initiatives lead to something that would count as a completely new technique. Because improvements are achieved by gradual refinement of existing techniques or the importation of something that has worked in another area, surgeons are often averse to randomization, and the nature of surgery means that neither they nor the patient can be blinded as to treatment or non-treatment. This does not rule out the possibility of randomized controlled trials but it does mean that creative alternatives or modifications to standard paradigms have to be found. The author advocates an Hippocratic approach which makes maximum use of careful observation and documentation, systematic review, and, where possible, statistically sound comparisons to evaluate new treatment.

INTRODUCTION

Surgeons are craftspeople with a foundation of medical science. Like all manual or technical artisans they fashion techniques to intervene in situations which need a skilful hands-on approach to care. This strength of surgery is also a weakness when it tries to map itself carefully on the grid of scientifically proper medical innovation with its rigorously controlled methods of comparative analysis. Several requirements for that methodology are sometimes hard to meet—for unavoidable reasons to do with the nature of the data and because of the constraints imposed by the surgeon's orientation towards benefiting by tried and tested techniques learnt from mentors and constituting a corpus of received knowledge.

There exists a well-established protocol for the introduction of new drug treatments in neurology and almost every area of medicine, but for surgical or other innovations no such mechanism is in place. Jennett (1986) notes several of the special difficulties posed by the evaluation of new operations, including maintaining blindedness in a trial (the blindedness problem); the effect of surgical skill (the varying skill problem); the generalizability of results from a centre of innovation and excellence (the generalization problem); and, the lack of knowledge about the costs and benefits of comparable existing techniques (the comparability problem).

There are several types of scenario that pose problems for the ethical surgeon. The first is when a tried and tested treatment is introduced to a new clinical setting. The second is when the surgeon adopts a novel use for an established treatment or technique. The third is when a health care professional devises a modification of an existing treatment. The fourth is when a health care professional invents a new approach to a problem. And the fifth is when a serendipitous discovery in relation to the treatment of one or more patients culminates in the development of an innovative treatment.

The first situation is very common. It does not cause any special concern and, in fact, goes on all the time as a result of technical notes in the literature and conference discussions of techniques in neurosurgery. The major issue that can arise in relation to tried and tested techniques being adopted in a new setting is the effect on morbidity and mortality of the inexperience of the operator and setting and therefore the generalization problem. The main ethical issue posed in this regard is the level of risk and benefit that should be communicated to patients in order to get informed consent to the treatment. Should the going rates at the best centres be communicated to the patient, knowing that the site at which the patient is treated may not live up to those figures? Here as elsewhere the patient should be given a clear view of the situation, the reasons why the new treatment is thought promising, and the fact that it is new to this centre.

Brian Jennett, in his discussion of high technology medicine, notes that the problems of surgical skill and the take-up of a new technique also create special difficulties in relation to the timing of assessment for new technologies because 'most series show a decline in mortality and morbidity as experience is gained' (1986, p. 95). I later argue that this factor proves to be crucial in obtaining ethically defensible informed consent to such a procedure and is just one further complication in relation to the other types of situation where innovative treatment is at stake.

The remaining situations all involve something being tried for the first time anywhere and raise a series of common issues which can be considered together. We can bring them into focus if we consider the treatment of Mr H.

> Mr H has been referred to a neurosurgical service with headaches, stiff neck, pains in the shoulders and arms, and occasional tingling in the left arm. He had lost a great deal of time off work with these complaints and was about to lose his job. Mr H is shown his MRI scan and the appearances which suggest a narrowing at C4,5, C5,6, and C6,7. His surgeon, call him Dr G, offers him a decompressive operation to the stenotic section of the cervical spine. There are several techniques for doing this but Dr G recommends a laminoplasty technique in which the

neural arches of C4, C5 and C6 will be bent backwards so as to create more room at the affected levels. He explains that his method of doing this involves the use of a locally developed innovation in which a Teflon and titanium device is used to maintain the expanded canal dimensions. There are no studies involving other centres which show the efficacy of this device.

As we consider the case of Dr G, we ought to remind ourselves of the Hippocratic injunctions about medical knowledge which were somewhat less rigid than the current fundamentalism of the prospective randomized controlled double blind trial. Hippocrates stressed the need for careful investigation of what nature throws up in the course of clinical practice with a refusal to be biased by pre-formed theories. 'Physicians', the writings claim, 'compare the present symptoms with similar cases they have seen in the past, so that they can say how cures were effected then' (p. 142). We shall see that this need for systematic observation is going to be important for reflective surgical practice.

JENNETT'S PROBLEMS AND MR H

Mr H poses, in a sharp and focused way, the major clinical problems of innovative treatment raised by Jennett; the blindedness problem, the varying skill problem, and the comparability problem all lurk beneath the surface of this consultation as well as problems about consent, the need for monitoring, the place of controlled trials, and the nature of surgery as a cumulative art with its own internal, even technical, values. Here the indications for which Mr H is being offered surgery are controversial and the device that Dr G is proposing to use is a local invention and has not been widely tested. Even if Dr G is a skilful surgeon and does his operations well, he cannot be blinded as to their having been done when he assesses their results and he may not have thought out how he will compare his technique with other possible approaches. We must therefore ask whether Dr G should offer Mr H this intervention and, if he does so, how should the technique he is proposing to use be regulated and evaluated from an ethical and scientific point of view?

To explore these and other issues which have a more general bearing on the development and introduction of new surgical techniques given the difficulties identified by Jennett, I pose a number of questions that an ethics committee ought to ask if they become aware of this innovative practice by Dr G (perhaps because he seeks their advice).

IS THIS A MODIFICATION OF AN ACCEPTED TREATMENT OR AN ALTERNATIVE?

There has been a gradual shift from laminectomy to laminoplasty world-wide among surgeons operating on the cervical spine. The reasons for this are not always well presented but the consensus seems to be that traditional laminectomy has a number of disadvantages (Herkowitz, 1988), such as development of swan neck deformity due to loss of spinal column support posteriorly (Sim *et al.*, 1974); late neurological progression in up to 60% of patients (Crandall and Gregorius, 1977; Yonenobu *et al.*, 1992); and, recurrence of stenosis due to dense fibrosis of the posterior operation site (Kimura *et al.*, 1995).

One might argue that these are all relatively unsupported beliefs if one applies strict evidential criteria to all clinical decisions, but throughout the practice of surgery there is a strong presupposition that standard treatment should be defined by a consensus of practising surgeons. In fact this is not totally irrational as the techniques of surgery require that you actually set out to correct a certain anomaly and achieve a result that looks anatomically better than the state you began with—pressure is relieved, distortion is corrected, pathological tissue is removed and so on. Given that there is a task to be done, and that initial attempts to do it are probably going to be refined over cumulative experience to the point where the surgeon does the job safely and well, there is likely to be a great deal of growth and development of best practice or best technique and relatively few major departures or new initiatives. It then becomes a question of degree as to whether a modification of an existing technique requires a total re-evaluation as distinct from a potentially revisionary re-examination of the practice as a whole.

These facts make it understandable that a surgeon such as Dr G might do a certain kind of operation—here posterior decompression of a compressed cervical spinal cord, in a certain way, here laminoplasty—and has come to the belief that it is superior in technical terms over his previous practice but has neither good evidence that standard practice is clearly beneficial nor, by implication, that his modification is a genuine improvement (in anything more than intraoperative technique). There are, in fact, a number of ways of doing cervical laminoplasty operations (Naito *et al.*, 1994), none of which has ever been demonstrated in a well-designed clinical trial to be superior either to laminectomy or to conservative management. One of the most common methods used is the open-door technique (Satomi *et al.*, 1994). This technique increasingly is done using a bone graft to avoid the problem of the lamina reverting to its stenotic position and the condition recurring (Baba *et al.*, 1996). Some surgeons have been concerned about the bone grafting technique most commonly used in open-door laminoplasty and have introduced other fixation techniques (Frank and Keenan, 1994). The device used by Dr G is an example of something produced as a result of the same kind of response—the desire to do what seems to be a technically superior operation. Dr G's device replaces the bone graft but does not fix the spinal laminae in place. It therefore differs in important respects from tried and tested techniques for this kind of surgery although it has been introduced in the same way as most modifications of surgical operations.

WHY WAS THIS MODIFICATION INTRODUCED?

Dr G noticed that the bone graft technique incorporated no safeguard against potential instability of the graft and worried that a shift in position would compromise the spinal cord. He also noticed that the most painful part of the operation was often the graft donor site on the iliac crest. His further worry was that the posterior fusion of several levels of the cervical spine would lead to painful symptoms and loss of cervical spinal function, a worry echoed by other authors (Hamburger, 1995).

After he had designed a device, called a CG clip, with the help of an engineer who was an ex-patient, he noticed that the proposed modification might have several advantages: the device was more stable than the bone graft; he did not require a fusion to maintain the contours of the expanded canal; and the device avoided the problem of donor site pain.

With these advantages in mind an early stainless steel prototype was used on a patient who had been fully informed of the innovative nature of the technique and offered the benefit of a different specialist opinion. This was a success; there was minimal postoperative morbidity and good relief of symptoms. It was some time before a further suitable case presented itself but the same technique was offered with the same provisions and the case went equally well. It was at this point that it began to look as if he had on his hands an innovative treatment which needed more systematic study.

WAS A PROSPECTIVE RANDOMIZED CONTROLLED TRIAL DONE?

At this stage Dr G had a problem, hinted at but not explored in any detail by Jennett. A prospective randomized controlled trial (PRCT) requires the investigator to be in an equipoise condition. Equipoise exists when the investigator has no valid reason to believe that entering the patient into one or other of two treatments will confer any advantage. She can therefore, with good scientific and clinical conscience, say to a potential participant that there is nothing to recommend one treatment arm over the other. Dr G was not quite in this position. At this stage, he accepted the general neurosurgical consensus that long segment (more than three segments) stenosis causing cervical spondylotic myelopathy (CSM) was best treated by surgery rather than conservative means as was the practice of all his fellow specialists. Now it may be that all his fellow specialists, were their practice to be subjected to the cold light of the best possible evidence, would be proved wrong in their conviction. It is true that a critical examination of the literature does not provide incontrovertible or even sound evidence that surgery is the best treatment for this condition. But this question should be subject to a much larger randomized controlled trial of surgical decompression versus non-surgical management rather than something Dr G would do on his own using his limited pool of patients. He also needs to think of the consequences of not treating his patients according to academically accepted best practice on the basis of a rational but minority view about the lack of adequate evidence for the benefits of surgery in this condition. He is therefore, it seems, justified in leaving the final decision about surgery to the patient, having explained the likely success rate (approximately 60% he believed) and the uncertainties, risks, and rationale (empirical as it is) of surgery. Therefore he could not do a PRCT of CG clip laminoplasty versus no treatment because he genuinely believed that standard surgical practice meant that surgery was necessary. Hence, the treatment arm constituted the only defensible treatment if a patient is symptomatic to the extent that he is actively contemplating surgery. It is obvious that the comparability problem is going to loom large in assessing a surgical innovation such as that proposed by Dr G.

Perhaps, at this stage, he should revert to cervical laminectomy in a control treatment arm. This also seems an odd requirement in that he has become convinced by the literature, the consensus among his colleagues in major centres where a lot of such surgery is done, and his own experience with two patients who had had that operation that the disadvantages already described and increasingly recognized among fellow surgeons were real, although he does know of neurosurgeons who continue to do laminectomies. He had already performed several laminoplasties using the standard open-door technique with and without bone grafting and had noticed that in some cases there was recurrent stenosis of the spinal canal, although it was unclear that this had caused significant morbidity. It would therefore be conceivable to use a bone graft laminoplasty as the control arm of a trial. But equipoise failed here also for reasons already rehearsed: namely, there is considerable pain associated with the bone graft donor site in a significant number of people; there is no intrinsic stability in the bone graft operation; and, his new procedure takes on average one and a half hours less than other types of laminoplasty.

If it is beyond dispute that this new technique needs evaluation in a relatively objective way, what kind of trial is suitable? It is unclear what sort of PRCT would be indicated without a careful examination of the credentials of existing treatments and how they have been established.

WHAT IS KNOWN OF THE EXISTING TREATMENT'S EFFICACY?

There are two aspects to this question in the present case.

(1) What are the data relating to the existing or currently best treatment of cervical spondylosis?
(2) What are the recognized indications and are there any reasons why Dr G might be justified in departing from them?

A wide range of results have been reported for the surgical treatment of cervical spine myelopathy (CSM). Epstein and Epstein's comprehensive review (1989) showed a mean 'success' rate of 72% for all techniques. Another review showed success rates ranging from 33% to 85% (Rowland, 1992). There are several difficulties with such data. The first is that indications for surgery differ between series, and are not always defined in the papers. A second is that outcome measures vary from study to study and are often not reported in any detail. Third, the assessment before and after surgery was often carried out by the surgeon doing the procedure or his team and therefore there is in many cases a reason for bias in the results. Furthermore, often we are not told of inclusion and exclusion criteria for such a surgical series.

The issue of defining indications can only be resolved by carefully structured clinical trials, but there is usually a gradation between absolute and relative indications. Absolute indications would generally include progressive myelopathy with loss of upper and/or lower limb function but may also include evidence of clear-cut neurological deficit, whether stable or progressive, and pain sufficient to compromise the normal function of the individual in day-to-day life. Pain is normally a relative indication and like all relative indications, in the most ethically informed hands, the decision to operate or not will rest with the patient once the prospect of operative success has been outlined as clearly as it can be.

The problem of variability in the outcome measures may eventually be solved by the use of standardized scales. The Japanese Orthopedic Association published the widely used JOA scale (1994). This scale takes account of upper and lower limb function, urinary symptoms and overall performance status. Unfortunately, facility with chopsticks is used in the assessment of upper limb function. There are no readily apparent analogues amongst the activities of daily living in Western countries. No doubt with this weakness in mind, the Neurosurgical Cervical Spine Scale (NCSS, Kadoya, 1992) was developed. It consists of a similar functional status assessment to that of the JOA scale, but without the reference to chopsticks or urinary function. Despite the applicability of the NCSS in both Western and Eastern contexts, the scale has not yet been widely adopted. For this reason it is quite difficult to assess just how much good we are doing, for what symptoms and which types of patients, by operating on CSM.

Thus the decision as to which symptoms ought to occasion the patient being offered surgery is entirely unclear on the basis of existing evidence. This is an unhappy situation. In fact, in the case of Mr H, the patient was offered surgery for unconventional indications as the result of an Hippocratic process. Hippocrates remarked, 'Medicine has for long possessed the qualities necessary to make a science. These are a starting point and a known method according to which many valuable discoveries have been made over a long period of time.' (Lloyd, 1978, p. 71). He goes on to describe how careful observations of clinical practice are accumulated over time until conclusions can be drawn as to which methods are effective and which not. In the case of headache and neck stiffness from cervical spondylotic stenosis (CSS), the path was classically Hippocratic.

At first Dr G was doing only the standard techniques but he gave patients the chance to talk about what their disease and their operation had meant to them. He began to get certain surprises. He noticed, for instance, that a number of them spontaneously reported resolution of tension-type headaches after cervical discectomy. For some patients this was the most significant single change as a result of surgery. He began to regard it as a significant part of the pattern of indications for surgery. Second, he began to notice that those patients with MRI proven long segment CSS were particularly troubled by headaches and that in those for whom a laminoplasty had been done for other more conventional reasons the resolution of headaches had been their major quality-of-life-affecting outcome. Eventually this pattern of morbidity and its resolution after surgery became so compelling that patients who wanted an operation mainly in the hope of getting rid of their headache were offered it with due warnings about the uncertainties and their entitlement to an alternative opinion (quite possibly differing from his own). Increasingly he found that patients were referred as 'domino' cases: they or their doctor had heard of somebody with a similar syndrome who had been dramatically relieved. We therefore have to ask what, from an ethical point of view, he should do at this point. Obviously there are a number of people who seem to have had a significant change in morbidity and functional status by opting for a relatively novel operation for controversial reasons. He cannot therefore, in service of his Hippocratic duty to benefit his patients, just ignore his own observations. But it seems, at the very least, that he should monitor his cumulative results to check for comparability to existing alternative treatments in terms of safety and efficacy so that he takes reasonable steps to ensure that he does not violate his duty to do no harm. It also seems that, where he has noted a surprising fact, the hypothesis that it is truly related to surgery ought to be submitted to rigorous statistical testing.

The first of these measures—a monitor of cumulative results—was done after 24 cases had been treated by him and another surgeon. The figures showed that the CG clip had similar results to other series in which patients had had posterior spinal surgery for CSS and CSM. The prima facie results therefore suggested that safety and efficacy were acceptable. Further questions must then arise and the question of the non-standard indications needs to be thoroughly investigated.

IS NEW MORBIDITY AND MORTALITY LIKELY?

This is obviously an important issue and bears on another observation in the Hippocratic corpus whereby we are enjoined to reason about a course of clinical management and, by reasoning, approximate to full knowledge of what we are doing (Lloyd, 1978, p. 77). In the present case, reasons have already been given why the modification was thought likely to be more sound than its competitors in that it improved operative technique by being more effective and causing less morbidity. From the observation of the initial series we can add to the technical appraisal the fact that there is no evidence that any adverse effects or deficiencies have come to light. This implies that questions of informed consent become extremely important in an ethical appraisal of Dr G's advice.

HAVE THE PATIENTS BEEN INFORMED?

This is the single most important ethical consideration. Once the scientific and clinical information has shown that the treatment seems to be at least as good as conventional treatment, the patients must know their options and how the advice that they are being given relates to a representative body of medical opinion. Many clinicians, and surgeons in particular, are bad at this in that they will make up their mind about a preferred mode of therapy and not inform the patient about uncertainties or options for treatment in other ways. In the end the patients must be empowered to make their own decisions where clinical certainty is not to be had or even where clinical facts are relatively clear but do not unequivocally point to one outcome—mastectomy versus lumpectomy in breast cancer for instance.

Dr G has obviously done this, and his patients seem to have become participants in designing their own treatment regimen and monitoring their own outcomes. Such a partnership allows medical innovation to proceed in a very fruitful way because the patients feel permitted to contribute their own observations no matter how odd or unusual these seem to be. Any researcher who does not avail himself or herself of this rich source of truly Hippocratic data is cutting off the branch on which advances in medicine have hung for over 2000 years.

However, the possible weakness of this position is the vulnerability of patients and the unequal power relationships in the clinical encounter. Obviously the partnership model tends to counteract this effect but it means that certain further questions must be asked.

DOES DR G HAVE A FINANCIAL INTEREST IN THE TECHNIQUE?

This question presses because of the difficulties of deriving clear evidence against agreed standards of practice in surgery. It is not likely that there will be vast differences in morbidity and mortality between different ways of doing the same thing, and therefore the reasons why an individual surgeon might tend towards one technique rather than another are open to all kinds of influences. A strong financial incentive to do things in a certain way, perhaps in a way that brings advantages to himself, would therefore be important in the considerations of an ethics committee. The fact that Dr G might be a co-inventor would constitute an important reason to insist on some kind of independent monitoring of results of surgery as the problem of non-blindedness would then be compounded by a very significant potential source of bias to slant the interpretation of outcomes in favour of the technique. The existence of such an interest does not constitute an absolute reason to refuse Dr G any role in the study of the device but it does give good reason to insist on objective and fairly robust standards of impartiality in the gathering and assessment of data about the operation.

HAS AN ETHICS COMMITTEE REVIEWED THE TECHNIQUE?

It is important that a competent body comprising both patients and professionals review innovative treatments. There needs to be a balance on such a committee because the patient's voice is at least as important as the professional voice on such issues and can offer an important check to either of two competing tendencies.

The first tendency is a relatively crusty and reactionary reversion to received wisdom in areas where innovation may well offer new possibilities at the expense of established theory; the case of gastric ulceration and *Helicobacter pylori* springs to mind. The second is a rather bullish enthusiasm for new technology which may be costly and relatively untried in its proposed application. The case of invasive cavernous sinus surgery springs to mind here.

The ethics committee should assure itself not only that these two sources of bias have been removed from their discussion but also that the surgeon involved is competent and held in good regard by other specialists in his area of specialty. This would presumably include evidence that the technique had been presented at professional meetings and/or conferences and been subject to review by his colleagues.

In New Zealand, unlike many other countries, there are well-established ethics committees with 50% lay and 50% professional membership. They are required to review both treatment and research. Such a committee was consulted about this new treatment. The committee made a decision to allow the treatment to proceed on the condition that patients would know exactly the respects in which the treatment was innovative, be aware that they could opt for conventional treatment, and that the committee would hear of any unusual or adverse outcomes. This decision obviously strikes a balance between recognizing the need for clinical management to be innovative and making sure there are adequate safeguards for patients.

HAVE THE ETHICS COMMITTEE'S REQUIREMENTS BEEN MET?

The requirements were met in part by the review of the first 24 cases but it is clear that this preliminary review based on careful clinical follow-up was insufficient to answer any but the most elementary questions about safety and efficacy.

WILL THERE BE MONITORING?

Most ethics committees are equipped to do regular checks of proposals submitted to them, at least in terms of self-report by the investigators. The facility for spot checks of adherence to the protocol by investigators is not so widely found and is much more costly and time-consuming to implement. It seems that a mechanism for spot checks by somebody independent of any involvement in the actual treatment, particularly for new treatments or new investigators, and especially when there may be financial or other interests involved, is one that should be fostered. It is interesting, however, that this treatment, perhaps even in contradistinction to conventional treatments, is being offered according to an informed choice or empowerment model of consent. Ideally, all treatment regimens should allow the patient some access to evidence based information about their treatment options, and the requirements for a regular audit of practice should be a minimum for surgical units.

IS A RANDOMIZED CONTROLLED TRIAL INDICATED?

The difficulties with PRCT for surgical techniques have already been canvassed but I shall briefly review them.

The surgeon has usually introduced the modification or new technique for a good set of reasons, as in the case under discussion. This implies that he is not in an equipoise condition: he cannot sincerely say that there is no reason to prefer either of the two possible alternatives because the lower morbidity, operating time, and the technical superiority of the modified procedure are all facts which favour the innovation over the alternatives.

The fact that any given surgeon will have his own or her own favoured technique for a procedure means that the best comparisons that can be achieved are usually prospective contemporaneous trials of non-randomly allocated patients receiving different treatments or comparisons between historically distinct retrospective series. Both of these present problems in that they fail to control for the differing skills of different surgeons and they may fail to achieve comparability on other measures such as case mix and peri-operative management.

The idea of blinding and placebo control is not really appropriate in surgery because placebo operations are not ethically acceptable.

Some of these problems can be ameliorated by careful attention to case mix in the series compared, correction of morbidity and mortality statistics in retrospective series by using a marker procedure of similar difficulty to that contemplated, standardized questionnaires and instruments for measuring indications and outcomes, and careful assessment of diagnostic and other parameters used in the series. They are also addressed in part by the uncertainty principle referred to by Lindley and Warlow in Essay 7. This provides for the doctor to be genuinely reflective about the standard of evidence and, where he acknowledges uncertainty, or the evidence is inconclusive about the best treatment for this patient, to seek to be part of a well-designed trial to address that uncertainty. This orientation is clearly needed in many areas of surgery.

WHAT SHOULD DR G SAY TO MR H?

If we take seriously the model of consent and medical advice in which a patient is empowered to make intelligent choices about his or her own care, it follows that Dr G cannot deny Mr H treatment on the basis of a unilateral medical decision—he must outline the options available, which include his CG clip technique.

This being so, Dr G must portray as accurately as he can the relative merits of different options and the morbidity to be expected with each. He must also inform Mr H about the uncertainties surrounding innovation and offer an alternative, independent, and perhaps more conventional opinion from another specialist.

When all is said and done, Dr G has a prima facie duty to do the operation that he has reason to believe is the most cost-effective and the least likely to cause complications. If this implies that he must use his new technique then so be it. If he does use his technique in patients like Mr H, he is bound to audit his results carefully and attempt to do some kind of valid clinical comparison that will yield the best possible evidence as to the relative scientific merits of his and other techniques.

The fact that he does not have a satisfying theoretical basis for his observations about the beneficial effects of his technique on cervical spondylotic headache is no barrier to doing the procedure on empirical grounds as theory often lags behind data and, if we are being scientific, that is as things should be. However, in an area where the results of surgery are partly assessed on the basis of quality-of-life criteria highly susceptible to all the biases that a PRCT is designed to eliminate, it seems that a PRCT is mandatory. We can now return to problems listed above: the blindedness problem, the surgical skill problem, and the comparability problem. Some of these are insuperable but that need not bar careful assessment of surgical innovations by use of a variety of methods which incorporate checks and balances (such as independent assessment, the use of the uncertainty principle, careful documentation of case mix, and objective assessments of outcome) against some of the sources of bias in clinical reports.

CONCLUSION

When we contemplate innovation and advance in a predominantly empirical enterprise such as surgery we must sometimes exercise our critical faculties to work towards filling in those areas of uncertainty and ignorance which abound in the messy world of clinical practice. We can be guided in our attempts to do this well by returning to the ancient sources of medical wisdom and relearning the value of Hippocrates' advice and reflections:

> I contend that the science of medicine must not be rejected as non-existent or ill-investigated because it may sometimes fail in exactness. Even if it is not always accurate in every respect the fact that it is able to approach close to a standard of infallibility as a result of reasoning, where before there was great ignorance should commend respect for the discoveries of medical science. Such discoveries are the product of good and true investigation, not chance happenings. (Lloyd, 1978, p. 77)

REFERENCES

Baba H, Chen Q, Uchida K, Imura S, Morikawa S and Tomita K (1996) Laminoplasty with foraminotomy for coexisting cervical myelopathy and unilateral radiculopathy. *Spine* 21:196–202.
Crandall P and Gregorius F (1977) Long term follow-up of cervical spondylotic myelopathy. *Spine* 2:139–146.
Epstein JA and Epstein NE. (1989) The surgical management of cervical spinal stenosis, spondylosis, and myeloradiculopathy by means of the posterior approach. In: *The Cervical Spine* (ed Cervical Spine Research Society), pp. 625–669. Philadelphia: Lippincott.
Frank E and Keenan TL (1994) A technique for cervical laminoplasty using mini plates. *British Journal of Neurosurgery* 8:197–199.
Hamburger C (1995) T-laminoplasty—a surgical approach for cervical spondylotic myelopathy. Technical note. *Acta Neurochirurgica* 132:131–133.
Herkowitz HN (1988) A comparison of anterior cervical fusion, cervical laminectomy, and cervical laminoplasty for the surgical management of multiple level spondylotic radiculopathy. *Spine* 13:774–780.
Japanese Orthopedic Association (1994) Scoring system for cervical myelopathy. *Journal of the Japanese Orthopedic Association* 68:490–503.
Jennett B (1986) *High Technology Medicine*. Oxford: Oxford University Press.
Kadoya S (1992) Grading and scoring system for neurological function in degenerative cervical spine disease—Neurosurgical Cervical Spine Scale. *Neurologia Medico-Chirurgica* 32:40–41.
Kimura I, Shingu H and Nasu Y (1995) Long term follow-up of cervical spondylotic myelopathy treated by canal-expansive laminoplasty. *Journal of Bone and Joint Surgery* 77:956–961.
Lloyd GER (1978) *Hippocratic Writings*. London: Penguin.
Naito M, Ogata K, Kurose S and Oyama M (1994) Canal expansive laminoplasty in 83 patients with cervical myelopathy. *International Orthopaedics* 18:347–351.
Rowland LP (1992) Surgical treatment of cervical spondylotic myelopathy: time for controlled trial. *Neurology* 42(1):5–13.

Satomi K, Nishu Y, Kohno T and Hirabayashi K (1994) Long term follow up studies of open-door expansive laminoplasty for cervical stenotic myelopathy. *Spine* **19**:507–510.

Sim FH, Suien HJ, Bickel WH and Janes JM (1974) Swan neck deformity following extensive cervical laminectomy. *Journal of Bone and Joint Surgery* **56A**:564–580.

Yonenobu K, Hosono N, Iwasaki M, Asano M and Ono K (1992) Laminoplasty versus subtotal corpectomy. A comparative study of results in multisegmental cervical spondylotic myelopathy. *Spine* **17**:1281–1284.

9

Who Should Receive, and Who Dispense, Expensive Treatments? The Example of Beta-Interferon

David Bates

ABSTRACT

This essay discusses the equitable introduction of new and expensive treatments. Costs of research and development tend to drive up the price of new medications. This is causing a particularly serious difficulty in neurology which abounds with previously untreatable chronic disorders, for which costs of pharmacotherapy have until now been low. The difficulty is compounded by the fact that many of the new treatments are of limited or even marginal efficacy. In some countries, such as the UK, local decision making has led to uneven availability of novel therapies. Both patients and professionals perceive that this is unfair. Wide international differences in prescribing practice exacerbate their sense of unease. By drawing attention to the patchy and restricted introduction of beta-interferon in the treatment of multiple sclerosis in the UK, this essay illustrates the ethical pitfalls in the prescription of costly novel agents.

INTRODUCTION

The advent of biotechnology and the development of novel medicines give grounds for optimism for the future management of many diseases currently regarded as incurable. The clinical neurologist sees many such patients with diseases that are neurodegenerative, neurogenetic or neuroinflammatory, which have long been regarded as incurable and usually untreatable. But the development of new therapies for conditions which are often only slowly progressive and for which there are no true animal models, while positive, also poses special problems for the therapies' assessment and evaluation. Biotechnology, and especially the production of active molecules by genetic manipulation of cells, tends to involve expensive manufacturing technique and clinical trials in chronic disease need to be prolonged, involve large numbers of patients, and frequently require ancillary investigations. The costs of development must be recouped and often results in the final product being extremely expensive. The problem of expensive medicines has always been more apparent in the non-surgical and non-oncological specialities and is particularly evident in neurology where a dearth of therapies for chronic degenerative and inflammatory diseases and a pervading nihilism about treatment has resulted in a discipline with very low therapeutic costs.

When curative treatments for motor neurone disease, the dementias, multiple sclerosis and the neurogenetic conditions become available they will be widely acclaimed, but when novel treatments can offer only partial effectiveness and are very expensive, clinicians and patients will have differing priorities. Decisions as to who shall receive the therapies and who prescribe them become of major importance.

WHO SHOULD RECEIVE EXPENSIVE THERAPIES?

The simplistic answer is that all of those likely to benefit from a novel therapy should be able to receive it. In the case of a new curative therapy this would include all patients with the identified disease. Most novel therapies, particularly in chronic conditions, are unlikely to be curative but rather will ameliorate the disease process. Therefore, perhaps, their usage should be limited to those most likely to benefit. The problem is how to determine those who are likely to benefit from a novel therapy. In most instances, since the therapy is brought into practice after controlled clinical trials which commonly include a carefully specified cohort of patients selected on the basis of age, sex, type of disease or those likely to show a significant change within the time span of the trials, it is suggested that new treatments should first be made available for similar patients. Authorities may recommend that the novel treatment initially be made available only to those patients identical to those involved in the pivotal trial and only when they fulfill the same rigid requirements as were defined for the trial cohort. This has a potential advantage for those involved in funding expensive treatment, in that it limits the availability of the therapy, but it inevitably places the onus for determining which patients fulfill the criteria on the individual physician. Two questions follow: who should define the criteria, whether they are those used in the trials or others?; and who will be the physician applying the criteria to the individual patient?

To some extent the criteria identifying which patients may be given novel treatments will be defined by the licensing authority. But these national bodies rarely specify precise requirements for the initiation of therapy, and although they are rigid in determining effectiveness and safety, they rarely assess comparative efficacy and instead provide a more general approach to the licensing of an individual product. The manufacturer will be required to define precisely the details of the license awarded, and consequently the criteria for patients who might be eligible, but cannot be expected to be proscriptive in the use of an agent and is likely to suggest, through marketing, advertising, medical news releases, financial reports and its representatives, that the therapy should be widely available.

So who can be expected to act as 'honest broker' and assimilate evidence upon which a reasonable and fair selection of patients for novel therapy can be made? Who should evaluate the evidence in 'evidence based medicine' (Kerridge *et al.*, 1998)? Logic would suggest that a national authority should be responsible for the definition of such criteria but most medicines control agencies, both in North America and Europe, have long felt that their role is to determine safety and efficacy rather than define the minutiae of prescribing. In those few countries, notably Australia and Scandinavia, where cost-effectiveness agencies exist, it is reasonable to expect them to define specific indications for the most expedient and cost-effective use of new medicines. The recently formed National Institute for Clinical Effectiveness in the UK may develop such a role.

In practice the majority of new therapies introduced to previously barren fields, and specifically new expensive therapies, are introduced after licensing through hospital consultants with the specific or tacit agreement of 'third party payers'—the insurers or the purchasers. Where funding for a new drug is uniform throughout a country this results in a reasonable equality of opportunity for individuals who might benefit from the drug. In those countries, like the UK, where there has been devolution of responsibility for aspects of health care down to small local authorities, the advent of novel therapies can result in divisiveness and marked inequality of provision. 'Prescription by postcode' cause patients and doctors to perceive inequality and consequently worry about ethical decisions (Department of Health, 1992). When local bodies, rather than a national organization, whether private or public, are expected to make decisions about availability of therapy for individual patients there is a potential for inequality of provision and a problem that inadequate experience, knowledge and information may manifest as local variation and be perceived as bias for or against an individual patient.

The process of devolution in health care presumably has as its goal the ultimate aim that every family practitioner or small local group will be responsible for their patients. If they are expected to decide the eligibility of individual patients for a novel therapy it will severely compromise their position as the advocate for their patient in respect of his disease and in support of his wish for treatment. The individual doctor or local practitioner group cannot effectively be both advocate for and judge towards the lone patient (Kassirer, 1998). An alternative would be to expect the local purchasers, the local or regional health authority, to be given the right to define which patients should be eligible for a new treatment. They cannot be expected to have the resources, statistics and expertise which are available to a national body, and they are inevitably more likely to be affected by local bias. The most ethical solution to the problem of defining which patients are eligible for a new and expensive therapy must be that the decision should be made by a national body which can assimilate all of the information from trials, consult the relevant experts, and interrogate both trialists and manufacturers. It should then be able to produce guidelines which, though not necessarily agreed by all physicians and certainly not accepted by all patients, could be reasonably administered by the individual doctor and adhered to by the individual patient.

The basis upon which such a national body might be expected to make decisions would include full information from clinical trials. They should have with the legal right to see and investigate all the original data, both from trials funded by pharmaceutical companies and those funded by academic bodies; none are necessarily free from bias or error. In addition to studying the overall trial results, assessors should be able to define cohorts or subgroups of patients expected to fare particularly well with the new therapy and those for whom no benefit can be expected. They might reasonably suggest methods of selecting patients, a protocol for monitoring, and a realistic time over which the new treatment should be assessed. They could also define criteria which could lead to it being withdrawn. Such a national body should also be able to determine when to require further trials of medication and ultimately to overrule the licensing authority and so prevent a licensed but clinically ineffective or cost-ineffective therapy from being prescribed or reimbursed.

The role of the patient in determining who shall be eligible for novel therapy is difficult. In many respects the patient is the single most important person in any disease process, a fact which is particularly evident in chronic diseases. Patients and their carers and relatives become very knowledgeable about their condition and learn from the media or the Internet much about perceived effectiveness of therapies. It is impracticable to allow the individual patient to be the decision maker with regard to novel therapies although the patient will always retain a veto. They should certainly be involved with their physicians in making the decision, even if only to recognize that a decision which they perceive as being against them is being made elsewhere. Patient groups, however, do have a role to play both in explaining indications and effects of therapies to their members and in acting as pressure groups to assist politicians in making executive and strategic decisions. Whether individual disease societies should be involved in discussions with local or national providers in determining the availability of novel therapies is a more difficult question but they should certainly be encouraged to make submissions to the relevant organizations prior to the decision-making procedure.

Pharmaceutical companies have an important facilitatory role in providing information to the licensing authority and to the funding bodies. They probably also have a role in helping politicians to formulate national policy but they should not have a role in determining which patient receives or is eligible for individual therapy. The arrival of new and expensive therapies has coincided, throughout the world, with new methods of providing information to patients. The ethical pharmaceutical industry used to regard its target as the medical profession, but with 'news' items in both the financial press and popular media on 'novel treatments' and with the use of websites related to specific disease processes there is increasing access by pharmaceutical companies to patients and carers to inform them about the potential for new treatments in chronic disease. Such information is important in raising public awareness of the chronic illness and in providing factual knowledge and hope to those who suffer from that disease, making them aware of possible therapies. But such news items are inevitably brief and often not wholly accurate. Although they may serve to bring to medical attention people with the specified illness, they cannot and should not be expected to modify the availability of the agent or to help in identifying those for whom the treatment should be available.

WHO SHOULD DISPENSE EXPENSIVE TREATMENTS?

One of the original concepts of the National Health Service (NHS) in the UK was that doctors should prescribe whatever agents were likely to benefit their patients. Originally the local doctor, possibly with specialist consultation, decided which drug should be used. Many of the agents prescribed were of limited efficacy and most of unknown cost. As medicine moved into the era of clinical accountability it became increasingly important that the doctor, whether locally or nationally, who made a decision about the availability of a therapy, assessed and understood the nature of its clinical efficacy. No one would want to prescribe an agent that was less clinically effective than another agent in the same condition, but what of those occasions where one disease is completely cured by a clinically effective drug but another disease is only palliated by one of lesser clinical efficacy? The second agent might reasonably be prescribed if it was the only therapy available for that condition, so that 'clinical efficacy' is a relative rather than an absolute criterion when comparing between disease states.

The problems inherent in comparing clinical efficacy between disease states are magnified when trying to compare cost-effectiveness of different drugs in different diseases. How can one compare the cost-effectiveness of a relatively cheap agent which totally relieves symptoms that would have lasted for 24 hours with one that partially relieves symptoms that would persist for years? Attempts can be made by the utilization of multiple assessment scales like the Nottingham Health Profile (Bowling, 1991) or from an evaluation of health state and duration of survival in the form of quality adjusted life years (QALY). It is then possible to determine a relative cost-effectiveness scale between treatments and diseases (Williams, 1985).

Having determined such rates of cost-effectiveness so far as possible, who shall be responsible for prescribing and for determining the availability of a drug; who will, in effect, be responsible for 'rationing'? It seems axiomatic that such decisions must be taken nationally; the local doctor, the local neurologist or consultant ought to be the patient's advocate if the patient decides that he or she wishes to take a novel therapy about which they have been informed. Their medical advisors at a local level should be able either to advise them that it will not be beneficial to them or explain that, although it might be potentially beneficial, that benefit has not been deemed worthy of support and reimbursement by the insurer, health service or government. If the local doctor or neurologist tries to explain to the patient that a drug which might potentially be of benefit to them is not potentially beneficial 'enough', then the patient ought to seek another counsellor who will be 'on their side'.

When, and if, novel therapies for neurological conditions are licensed and prescribable they should be prescribed by the neurologist, who will be responsible to the insurers or purchasers for the collection of data about the progress of the individual patient, the possible development of complications and subsequent decisions regarding cessation or change of therapy, which must be justified. When expensive new therapies are brought into use they must be carefully monitored and some attempt made over time to compare the progress of individual patients with historical controls. It would be unreasonable for a physician to make an important decision about the introduction of an expensive novel therapy but then to delegate assessment of its effect to others.

BETA-INTERFERON

The most appropriate recent example of the introduction of an expensive novel therapy in neurology is the advent of beta-interferon for patients with multiple sclerosis. The first interferon β was licensed for patients with acute remitting relapsing multiple sclerosis who fulfilled certain criteria of age, disability and frequency of attacks in the US in 1994 and in Europe in 1995. There are now three agents available; interferon β-1b and two makes of interferon β-1a. By the end of 1998 the proportion of patients with remitting-relapsing multiple sclerosis who were eligible to receive such therapy (estimated at about 10% of the total number of MS patients) who were actually receiving treatment was about 25% in the US, 15% in Australia, 7–10% in continental Europe and only 1% in the UK. If the North American physicians and patients are correct in their usage of the agent then the situation in the UK is indefensible and unethical, but if the UK usage is correct and appropriate then that in North America is inappropriate. Why is there such a difference?

The fact that interferon β has a clinical effect in multiple sclerosis cannot be doubted. There are now three large pivotal studies in patients with relapsing remitting multiple sclerosis from North America and Europe. Two show a statistically significant reduction of attack rate by about one-third, the third shows a similar trend. Two also show a reduction in disease progression and the third a similar but non-significant trend (IFNB Multiple Sclerosis Study Group, 1993; Jacobs *et al.*, 1996; PRISMS, 1998). MRI scan data from two of the trials show a remarkable reduction in new lesion formation and a reduction in the rate of increase of abnormal signal on T2 weighted images, the 'burden of disease', in patients treated with the agent (Paty and Li, 1993). Most people would accept that a one-third reduction in attack rate, together with evidence for reduction in severity of attacks and the objective findings of a lessening of need for hospital admission and steroid therapy is a significant clinical benefit. All would recognize that a delay in deterioration of one year over the three years of a trial was significant. Therefore physicians and patients alike must recognize that interferon β has an effect upon multiple sclerosis.

It follows that the difference in usage between various countries must relate to different views of cost-effectiveness, in other words an uncertainty in the minds of physicians, insurers and purchasers as to whether the difference established in the trials is worth the cost of $15 000 or £10 000 per patient per year. In the cost-conscious health service of the United States the answer has been a resounding 'yes', and in continental Europe and Australasia, notably in Scandinavia and Australia where cost-effectiveness committees supersede the licensing authorities, the drug is presumably thought to be cost-effective and is used. Why then is the UK different? In part, it is because neurologists in the UK have been made very conscious of expensive drugs. Letters from the NHS Executive in 1994 and 1995, before the agent was licensed, talked of 'limited clinical benefit' and the fact that the drug was 'likely to be extremely expensive'. Strategic reports from local health authorities warned 'unsurprisingly, early products appearing in previously barren fields are only very rarely, if ever, wonder drugs. Their effects may be marginal and manufacturers seek (to price) these products at a level to maximize their return.'

In addition, neurologists have been faced with the requirement for increased accountability; but accountability to whom? – Certainly not the patient. The perceived accountability is probably to their local Trust and ultimately through their purchasers to the health service (Charlton, 1999). In some areas local purchasers have chosen to refuse to purchase interferon β and one health authority has been taken to court by a patient over failure to provide treatment which had been recommended by a neurologist. In general however, patients, their carers, their societies, their neurologists and their primary care physicians have accepted a low level of use of the agent, presumably on the grounds of cost-effectiveness.

As one neurologist wrote in 1996, 'If β Interferon were as cheap as aspirin and had an established safety record then neurologists would almost certainly be willing to give it a try on the strength of the data currently available. Conversely, if it were the subject of a series of rigorous, independent clinical trials with unequivocal evidence of effective slowing of disability accumulation, then neurologists would prescribe it, even at the current enormous cost. Unfortunately it is neither, hence the fuss' (Mumford, 1996). The analogy to aspirin, though not intended by the author, is appropriate since, in numerous trials, aspirin has been shown to be effective in reducing, not preventing, the risk of stroke by about one-third. This is similar to the one-third reduction in the rate of progression in multiple sclerosis, yet aspirin is widely used by those same neurologists in the UK who are cautious about interferon β.

However, problems in introducing the novel, expensive and partially effective therapy interferon β during the past few years in the small cohort of patients with relapsing remitting disease who fulfilled the criteria of the original trials should change dramatically. The first study of interferon β-1b in patients with secondary progressive multiple sclerosis has been published (European Study Group, 1998) and the treatment is licensed in North America and Europe. The immediate change for the prescribers is that the potential number of people with multiple sclerosis now eligible for therapy rises from about 10% of the total population with the disease to over 50% of that population. The potential benefit of a delay in progression of disease of up to 12 months during the three years of the trial may still be considered by critics to be 'marginal' but the suggestion to the individual patient of a reduction in the rate of deterioration by one-third is likely to be prove extremely attractive. It seems inevitable that further rationing of available therapy will occur as the indications for novel and expensive therapies are widened, the main remaining ethical question now being only the basis upon which that rationing is established.

There is nothing wrong with a process of rationing for any service or therapy, but such rationing should be equitable throughout the country. The present concern in the UK, unlike the US, is that there is rationing of a medicine by area—prescribing by postcode. Furthermore, the altruism of neurologists in refraining from the use of a therapy may be admirable and ethically sound but it will fail if colleagues in other disciplines spend the monies saved by avoiding expensive neurological treatment in less cost-effective ways. In that scenario only the MS patients will lose, creating a most serious ethical dilemma.

CONCLUSIONS

The introduction of expensive, but only partially effective medicines into disease areas where no effective curative therapy exists will always be difficult. It is inevitable that there will be a conflict between the idealist who wishes to do everything that might benefit the patient and the realist who recognises that we cannot afford to do everything, particularly as the costs of 'normal' health care and 'marginal therapies' increase. Whatever our politicians and health care insurers protest, there is rationing of health care benefits and any cost-containment mechanism, either from managed care or from a national health service, will create difficulty for physicians and patients in recognising that not all that is possible is necessarily practicable. Despite the mantra of there being 'no rationing within the health service' most physicians and patients understand the limitations, but both groups will respond better and certainly be more able to accept the concept of rationing as it affects the individual if it is seen to be fair and equitable within a country or a society rather than a lottery, depending upon the area of abode or the whims of the local provider.

A comparison of the way in which interferon β has been introduced and used in North America, continental Europe and the UK offers a variety of potential planning systems. Some appear to be equitable; others, so far, do not.

REFERENCES

Bowling A (1991) *Measuring Health: A Review of Quality of Life Scales*. Milton Keynes: Open University Press.

Charlton BG (1999) The ideology of 'accountability'. *Journal of the Royal College of Physicians of London* **33**:33–35.

Department of Health (1992) *The Health of the Nation*. London: HMSO.

European Study Group on interferon β-1b in Secondary Progressive MS (1998) Placebo-controlled, multiple centre, randomised trial of Interferon β-1b in treatment of secondary progressive multiple sclerosis. *Lancet* **352**:1491–1497.

IFNB Multiple Sclerosis Study Group (1993) Interferon β-1b is effective in relapsing-remitting multiple sclerosis. *Neurology* **43**:655–661.

Jacobs LD, Cookfair DL, Rudick RA *et al.* (1996) Intramuscular interferon β-1a for disease progression in relapsing multiple sclerosis. *Annals of Neurology* **39**:285–294.

Kassirer JP (1998) Managing care—should we adopt a new ethic? *New England Journal of Medicine* **339**:397–398.

Kerridge I, Loe M and Henry D (1998) Ethics and evidence based medicine. *British Medical Journal* **316**:1151–1153.

Mumford CJ (1996) Beta interferon and multiple sclerosis: why the fuss? *Quarterly Journal of Medicine* **89(1)**:1–3.

Paty DW and, Li DK (1993) Interferon β-1b is effective in relapsing remitting multiple sclerosis. *Neurology* **43**:662–667.

PRISMS (1998) Randomised, double-blind, placebo-controlled study of interferon β-1a in relapsing/remitting multiple sclerosis. *Lancet* **252**:1498–1504.

Williams A (1985) The economics of coronary bypass grafting. *British Medical Journal* **291**:326–329.

10

Why and When May Treatment Be Enforced?

Tony Hope

ABSTRACT

There are situations when a neurologist needs to consider whether to restrain a patient or to enforce treatment. This may be because the patient poses a danger to himself or others, or because he is refusing beneficial treatment. The physician may be able to resolve the problem by explaining her own position to the patient and by trying to understand the patient's viewpoint. When this is not possible, the key issue is whether the patient is competent to decide his own health care. A competent adult can refuse even life-saving treatment. An incompetent patient should normally be treated according to his best interests. It is therefore important for physicians to be able to assess the relevant competence of their patients. This essay outlines a practical approach and applies it to a number of problematic cases.

INTRODUCTION

Physicians traditionally have been guided by a central ethic: to do what is best for their patients. In recent times this ethic has been dubbed 'the principle of beneficence' (Beauchamp and Childress 1979; Gillon, 1985). Liberal societies are concerned, at least in theory, with enabling citizens to make their own choices, free from coercion. In the clinical setting this perspective stresses the point that it is for patients to choose whether or not to accept the treatments on offer. This has been called 'the principle of respect for patient autonomy' (Beauchamp and Childress 1979; Gillon, 1985). Most of the time what patients want, and what physicians think is best, will coincide. What should physicians do, however, when they believe that a patient is making a choice which is significantly against his best interests? In this essay I consider situations in which the neurologist may face the question: should I enforce treatment against the patient's will? I begin with a quotation from Barbellion which reminds us that the patient's perspective can, quite reasonably, be at odds with that of the physicians. I then describe four clinical situations which are further discussed in the second half of the essay in the light of the relevant ethical and legal principles.

DIFFICULT CASES FOR THE NEUROLOGIST

On October 5th, 1918, WNP Barbellion, who was dying from multiple sclerosis, wrote in his diary:

> Some London neurologist has injected serum into a woman's spine with beneficial results, and as her disease is the same as mine, they wish to try it too. I may be able to walk again, to write etc., my life prolonged!
>
> They little know what they ask of me … They can never understand—I mean my relatives— what a typhoon I have come through, and just as I am crippling into port I have no mind to put to sea again! I am too tired now to shoulder the burden of Hope again. (Barbellion, 1984)

Modern neurologists encounter patients who refuse beneficial treatments. Consider the following four situations:

> Mr A is suffering from an acute confusional state that turns out to be due to systemic lupus erythematosus (SLE). Even after acute treatment he remains somewhat confused. The medical opinion is that he requires continuing treatment with steroids and cyclophosphamide. Although confused he clearly refuses consent for such continuing treatment. Should Mr A's doctor enforce treatment?
>
> Ms B is suffering from multiple sclerosis. She regularly sees Dr X, a consultant neurologist, in the outpatient department. She tells Dr X that if her multiple sclerosis continues to deteriorate she will kill herself. Should Dr X take any steps, including restraint, to prevent Ms B from carrying out this act?
>
> Mr C is 25 years old. He is addicted to opiates, and possibly to alcohol as well. He is brought into casualty with minor injuries following an attempt to set fire to the block of flats in which he lives. The casualty officer observes that he has nystagmus and calls in the neurologist. When the neurologist arrives Mr C is behaving aggressively and poses a danger to both himself and others. The presumed diagnosis is of acute confusional state, likely to be secondary to either drug intoxication or withdrawal. In order to carry out the investigations needed for definitive diagnosis, and in order to protect both himself and others, Mr C needs to be sedated.
>
> Ms D is in her early fifties. She has cervical cord compression presumed to be due to cervical spondylosis. The cord compression is leading to her becoming shaky on her legs. She is offered surgery in order to relieve the compression. She refuses the surgery saying that she is too scared to come into hospital. The expert view is that with surgery she stands a chance of returning to full mobility. Without surgery she may deteriorate and eventually become incontinent and die of repeated infections. Should Ms D's doctors enforce beneficial treatment on her?

PATIENT AUTONOMY

The right to patient autonomy, in the medical context, emerged as a legal doctrine in English law in 1767 in the case of Slater v. Baker and Stapleton (see

Faden and Beauchamp, 1986, p. 116). The judge said: 'It appears from the evidence of the surgeons that it was improper to disunite the callous without consent'. However, it is in the US that the legal doctrine of informed consent has developed. The classic statement was made in 1914 by Justice Cardozo in the case of Schloendoff v. Society of New York Hospital (211 NY 125 1914):

> Every human being of adult years and sound mind has a right to determine what shall be done with his own body; and a surgeon who performs an operation without his patient's consent commits an assault for which he is liable in damages.

This judgement, which has been effectively integrated into English law (Kennedy and Grubb, 1994; Montgomery, 1997), gives patients of 'sound mind' the clear legal right to refuse medical and surgical treatment. Such refusal is valid even if the patient is likely to come to serious harm as a result of the refusal. The importance of providing patients with information (informed consent) was stated in the US case of Salgo in 1957 (see Faden and Beauchamp, 1986). The patient suffered permanent paralysis following trans-lumbar aortography. The court found that physicians had the duty to disclose 'any facts which are necessary to form the basis of an intelligent consent by the patient to proposed treatment'.

VALID CONSENT

Three elements of valid consent are generally recognized, both in law and ethics (Montgomery, 1997):

(1) The person is **competent** (has capacity).
(2) The person is **informed**.
(3) The person gives consent **voluntarily** (is not coerced).

The key legal issue when a patient is refusing, or resisting, beneficial treatment is: does the patient have capacity? 'Capacity' is the legal term equivalent to the clinical concept of competence. In English common law, whereas a competent adult has the right to refuse any treatment, an incompetent patient should be treated in his best interests (Fig. 10.1).

THE COMPETENT PATIENT

It is part of a physician's duty of care to ensure that a competent patient is properly informed and free from coercion.

INFORMED CONSENT

From the legal point of view there are two types of information that need to be given: the general nature of the procedure; and, the main risks and benefits of the

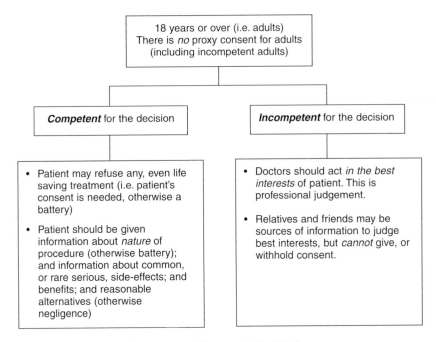

Figure 10.1   Consent in English law.

proposed treatment, compared with reasonable alternative treatments. This was established in the case of Sidaway v. Bethlem RHG (1985; see also Kennedy and Grubb, 1994). This general legal guidance leaves room for wide variation in practice. From the ethical point of view, the aim, in respecting patient autonomy, should be for the physician to provide the information to an extent, and in a form, that best helps the patient to decide (Hope, 1996). One extreme to avoid is the presenting of a mass of indigestible information that is done more to protect the doctor from legal action than to help respect the patient's autonomy. The other extreme is the paternalistic one, where the physician barely involves the patient in the decision-making process. Different patients, of course, will want to be involved in making the decision to different extents. The more the patient wants to leave the decision to the physician, the more important it is for the physician to find out what are the patient's values that are relevant to the decision.

VOLUNTARY CONSENT

The question of what counts as coercion in obtaining consent is far from straightforward. Clear coercion, such as the issuing of threats, is obviously wrong. The much more difficult issue is how much persuasion is allowable before that persuasion counts as coercion (Emanuel and Emanuel, 1992). One extreme view is that any persuasion is an infringement of patient autonomy. On this view a physician's job is to present the information on possible treatments in a neutral and unbiased way and to leave the patient to choose. There are, I think, three arguments against this purely informational approach to voluntary consent (Savulescu and Momeyer, 1997):

(1) It is not clear that this is what most patients would like. Therefore, respecting patient autonomy may be better served by not adopting this position.
(2) Such a neutral and unbiased method of presenting information is not, even in theory, possible.
(3) Far from conflicting with respect for autonomy, persuasion can enhance it. We test our beliefs through argument and discussion with others.

IS IT EVER RIGHT TO TREAT COMPETENT PATIENTS AGAINST THEIR WILL?

There are two possible reasons for justifying treatment of competent adults against their will. First, because the patient will come to harm unless treated; second because of risk of harm to others.

The legal and the ethical presumption is generally that treatment can not be forced on a competent adult. This position can, however, be questioned (Greaves, 1991). There are situations outside medicine where it is broadly accepted that best interests can override autonomy. The compulsory use of seat belts is one example.

But overriding autonomy in order to protect others is often contentious. Sometimes, the issue for doctors is whether this should be through compulsory medical treatment or whether it is a matter for the police (see below).

ASSESSMENT OF COMPETENCE (CAPACITY)

In the legal and ethical analysis of treating people against their will, a great deal depends on whether the patient is competent. The issue under discussion here is competence to make decisions about medical management. In some circumstances courts need to consider other types of competence, such as competence to stand trial.

Three broad approaches to the definition of competence can be distinguished (The Lord Chancellor's Department, 1997): by status; by outcome; and by function (specific). In the first approach competence would depend on what status the patient has: for example, a patient detained under the Mental Health Act, or a patient under the Court of Protection, might ipso facto be considered incompetent. This approach is rejected both by law and by most ethical analysis. An outcome approach examines the actual decision that a person makes. If the decision is silly, or irrational, then the person may, for that reason, be considered incompetent. The law does not endorse this approach. If a patient appears to be making a foolish decision, for example refusing beneficial treatment, the doctor needs carefully to assess the patient's competence. But to consider somebody incompetent purely on the grounds that their decision is wrong would be to fail to respect their autonomy.

The approach endorsed by both law and most ethical analysis is the functional approach. Common law has identified three components to capacity (Re C, 1994):

(1) the comprehending and retaining of information relevant to making the decision
(2) believing this information
(3) weighing the information in the balance and arriving at a decision.

In assessing competence, physicians need to clarify a patient's ability by applying each of these three components to the specific issue, or decision, in question. It would not be sufficient to provide a 'global' assessment, for example to the effect that a patient is suffering from dementia, with a mental test score of such and such. A consequence of the functional approach is that a patient may be competent to refuse to move into a nursing home, but incompetent to refuse antibiotics (or vice versa). The second component—believing the information—needs to be applied with care. The quality of information is not always high, and it is reasonable for patients to be sceptical of much clinical information. The main purpose of this component is to highlight the possibility that a patient who has the cognitive ability to understand and weigh up information may, nevertheless, be incompetent because of a delusion which interferes with believing key information. An extreme example is when a patient with a manic illness does not believe he will probably be killed if he jumps from a tenth floor window, because of the delusional belief that he can fly.

FACTORS AFFECTING COMPETENCE

Several factors of clinical relevance can interfere with the components of competence outlined above. Of particular importance are: cognitive (intellectual) ability; delusions and hallucinations; and significant mood disorder (depression; mania).

The analysis, outlined above, in English common law is particularly clear when applied to people with impaired cognitive ability. The difficult issue here is one of threshold. There is a presumption, in English law, in favour of capacity (The Lord Chancellor's Department, 1997). In other words, the degree of understanding should be set such that the vast majority of people are competent with regard to health care decisions. In the case of delusions and hallucinations this analysis implies that a person is incompetent only if the specific delusion or hallucination interferes with understanding, believing or reasoning about the issues specific to the decision (Re C, 1994). The analysis is at its weakest with regard to mood disorder. A depressed person may, for example, refuse beneficial treatment because, as a result of the depression, he does not care about his own welfare. Such a person may be able to understand, believe and, apparently, weigh up the issues. In common law, a depressed person could be considered incompetent on the grounds that the depression interferes with her ability to weigh up the issues and arrive at a decision. The Mental Health Act needs to be considered in this type of situation. It focuses not on competence but on mental disorder.

THE MENTAL HEALTH ACT

The Mental Health Act (MHA) may occasionally be relevant to compulsory treatment in neurology. Its use would normally require the involvement of a psychiatrist. There are three key points concerning the Mental Health Act:

(1) The Act is only relevant for a person with a mental disorder.
(2) The Act is only concerned with the treatment, or assessment, of the mental disorder. It is not relevant to treating physical disorders, unrelated to the mental disorder, of patients with a mental disorder.
(3) Being a Statute (Act), it 'trumps' common law, but only within its scope of reference.

The term **mental disorder** is defined as 'mental illness, arrested or incomplete development of mind, psychopathic disorder and any other disorder or disability of mind'. Dependence on alcohol or drugs is not sufficient grounds for mental disorder. The grounds for compulsory admission are that the person is suffering from a mental disorder warranting detention in hospital for assessment (or treatment), and that the detention is required for the person's health, or safety, or for the protection of others.

THE INCOMPETENT PATIENT

There are four theoretically possible approaches to making decisions about the health care of incompetent patients (Buchanan and Brock, 1989): best interests; substituted judgement; proxy; and advance directives.

Best interests
One approach for a physician faced with an incompetent patient is to ask the question: which plan of management serves the patient's best interests? This is the approach generally supported by English common law. It is part of the doctor's duty of care to judge best interests, and the physician is legally accountable for this judgement.

Substituted judgement
The criterion of substituted judgement asks the hypothetical question: suppose the patient were (magically) able to become competent, what treatment would

he choose? In order to try and answer this question the physician could use a range of evidence: reports of what the patient has said about this kind of situation in the past; the kind of general values which the patient held; and experience with other patients.

Proxy
An alternative approach is for a proxy to make decisions on behalf of an incompetent patient. Consider the case of Ms R, a 78-year-old widow who suffers from moderate to severe dementia (probably Alzheimer's disease). She fractures the neck of her femur in a fall. The orthopaedic surgeon strongly recommends surgery to repair the fracture. Ms R is not competent to give, or withhold, consent because of her cognitive impairment. Who, if anyone, should give consent (and sign the consent form) on behalf of Ms R? The answer in English law is that no-one can give consent. The decision is entirely in the physician's hands. This is because a central point in English law is that there is *no proxy consent for an adult*. Thus no person, not the patient's next of kin (not even a court) can either give or withhold consent. This is true even if Ms R is under the Court of Protection. The Court of Protection is concerned only with Ms R's possessions and has no power over her person. The possibility of nominating a health care proxy is currently under consideration (The Lord Chancellor's Department, 1997). Talking with the next of kin may be highly relevant in order to judge best interests, but the next of kin is not able to give or withhold the consent. A clear statement of this point was made in the case of Re F (1989): 'a doctor can lawfully give surgical or medical treatment to adult patients incapable of consenting provided the operation is in their best interests'.

Proxies play a much more important role in the US than in the UK. In the US, an appointed proxy acquires an additional legal authority to make decisions even if he or she is the next of kin.

Advance directives
See essay 14.

THE ROLE OF THE FAMILY

Doctors usually involve the families or close friends of patients not capable of making decisions for themselves. This is particularly important when doctors are considering enforcing treatment. There are five different types of information that a doctor may wish to gather from patients' relatives:

1. Evidence for explicit instructions which the patient had given to the family.
2. A general view of the patient's values.
3. Information on the patient's quality of life and likely quality of life.
4. The relatives' opinion of what is best for the patient.
5. The relatives' opinion as to what is best for themselves.

Relatives are often in a better position than doctors to judge these issues. If a particular management decision will go strongly against the interests of the relatives it is unlikely in the long run to be in the best interests of the patient. Furthermore, it is important to many people that they should not become a burden to their families (Nelson and Nelson, 1995). Whether a management decision which is not in the best interests of the patient should ever be carried out on the grounds that it is better for relatives is a moot point. In English law the courts would normally see the doctor's duty of care as directed to the patient only, and that duty would entail doing what is in the patient's best interests. However, if the patient's best interests require the relatives either to pay substantial sums (as may particularly be the case in the US) or to take much of the burden of care, then the relatives will de facto determine some of the key decisions.

THE CASES EXAMINED

An incompetent patient resisting beneficial treatment (case of Mr A)

In an acute situation (for example where a confused patient suffering from hypoglycaemia requires intravenous glucose) there is little doubt, both legally and ethically, that treatment can be enforced on an incompetent patient despite resistance. The patient should be treated in his best interests.

What is much more difficult is the situation illustrated by the case of Mr A (p. 111), where to treat the patient in his best interests requires frequent periods of conflict. In judging best interests the deleterious effect of these periods of conflict has to be put into the overall balance. Furthermore, there is an important practical issue. To hold someone down to administer glucose on a single occasion in hospital is relatively straightforward. To enforce oral treatment several times a day by care staff visiting in the person's home may either be impossible or an unreasonable imposition on care staff.

In coming to a decision the following points may help:

(1) Try and clarify what, all things considered, is in the patient's best interests.
(2) Try and answer the question of whether it is possible to get an idea of what the patient would have wanted.
(3) Involve in the discussion relevant other professionals and close friends or relatives.
(4) Where the decision is difficult it may be valuable to pursue one line of management for a period of time and see how it works out.
(5) Make use of opportunities, for example periods when the patient is not resisting treatment.
(6) The fact that the patient is incompetent may justify overriding his resistance, if this is the only effective way of acting in his best interests.

The apparently competent person threatening suicide (case of Ms B)

A competent Jehovah's Witness can refuse life-saving treatment. Does it therefore follow that a competent person threatening suicide cannot be prevented from carrying out the threat? There are two differences between these situations: first, that the desire to commit suicide may be part of a depressive illness; second, that it may be an acute reaction to an event and therefore not a stable decision. Buchanan and Brock (1989) argue that if a decision is not stable this may be grounds for considering the patient to be incompetent.

It is important for the neurologist to consider depressive disorder and, if necessary, seek a psychiatric opinion. Compulsory admission to treat this disorder may be justified under the Mental Health Act. The problem for neurologists is likely to occur when there is no clear depressive disorder and when the person's suicidal thoughts are likely to remain for a considerable period. The two theoretical possibilities are to detain the patient for a long time or to provide voluntary outpatient support. The former does not seem desirable in the case of Ms B. It would effectively make her a prisoner, potentially for the rest of her life. Nor is it likely to be legally acceptable. A patient can only be detained against her will by two methods: either under the Mental Health Act, in which case the person must be suffering from a mental disorder; or under the common law doctrine of necessity. In the latter case the person would need to be judged incompetent to refuse treatment. Furthermore, it is unlikely that the courts would be happy for someone to be detained against her will for a substantial length of time under common law. Perhaps all that Dr X can do in this case is to try and establish a supportive relationship with Ms B and to see her regularly, providing full supportive services on an outpatient basis.

The incompetent person requiring sedation (case of Mr C)

If, as seems to be the case with Mr C, the patient is clearly incompetent to decide his own health care, then the doctor should do what is in the patient's best interests. These would probably best be served by sedation followed by investigations carried out within a safe environment. Indeed it may be negligent for a doctor to allow Mr C to come to harm through not carrying out the necessary investigations.

A competent person who is making a silly decision (case of Ms D)

The first step when faced with a patient who is making an apparently silly decision is to find out her reasons. She may simply be wrongly informed or have had an experience that is unnecessarily dominating the decision. Discussing this openly and correcting any false information may solve the problem. It is legitimate, in my view, to try and persuade the patient of the foolishness of the decision. I have argued above that this respects, rather than overrides, autonomy. If the patient's reasons seem strange, then the physician needs to assess competence and consider the possibility of mental disorder.

However, the fact that the person is making a foolish decision, does not, by itself, provide grounds for declaring the person incompetent. Independent grounds are required. A competent adult who is not suffering from a mental disorder has, in the end, the right to make her own decision. The case of Ms D probably falls within this category.

It can be helpful for clinicians faced with a patient making an apparently foolish decision to adopt a structured approach, such as the following:

(1) Try and understand patients' reasons. Correct false information.
(2) Carefully evaluate alternative plans of management, their pros and cons.
(3) Assess competence in making the decision.
(4) Assess for mental disorder.
(5) Assess root causes of the foolish decision and address if possible.

The patient who is a danger to others

One of the most difficult situations that can face a doctor is when a patient constitutes a danger to other people. The steps in analysing this situation are:

(1) Is the patient suffering from a mental disorder? If so, seek psychiatric advice.
(2) Is the patient suffering from an acute confusional state? If so, restraint and treatment may be justified under common law.
(3) Is the patient a danger to others because of acute drug intoxication (and especially alcohol)? The Mental Health Act would rarely be used in this situation. If it is not possible to keep the person and others safe within the hospital then security staff or the police should be involved.
(4) Is the person fully competent? If so, then the police are likely involved already. If the person has a medical condition that also requires treatment then this would need to be undertaken in collaboration with the police. Other hospital patients should not be put at risk through the management of a patient who is a danger to others.

CONCLUSION

One of the most difficult situations for physicians is when they are uncertain whether they should enforce treatment or restrain a patient's freedom. Physicians need to know how the common law approaches the issue of enforcing treatment and restraining patients who may be a danger to themselves or others. They also need to know when the Mental Health Act could be relevant. However, good communication and a thoughtful approach to the ethical issues are the most important aspects of the doctor's approach.

Acknowledgements
I would like to thank Judith Hendrick and the editors, Adam Zeman and Linda Emanuel, for their very helpful comments on a previous version of this chapter.

REFERENCES

Barbellion WNP (1984) *The Journal of a Disappointed Man*, p. 321. London: The Hogarth Press.

Beauchamp TL and Childress JF (1979) *Principles of Biomedical Ethics*. New York: Oxford University Press.

Buchanan AE and Brock DW (1989) *Deciding for Others: The Ethics of Surrogate Decision Making*. Cambridge: Cambridge University Press.

Emanuel EJ and Emanuel LL (1992) Four models of the physician-patient relationship. *Journal of the American Medical Association* **267**: 22–29.

Faden RR and Beauchamp TL (1986) *A History and Theory of Informed Consent*. New York: Oxford University Press.

Gillon R (1985) *Philosophical Medical Ethics*. Chichester: John Wiley & Sons.

Greaves DA (1991) Can compulsory removal ever be justified for adults who are mentally competent? *Journal of Medical Ethics* **17**: 189–194.

Hope T (1996) *Evidence-Based Patient Choice*. London: King's Fund.

Kennedy I and Grubb A (1994) *Medical Law*. London: Butterworths.

The Lord Chancellor's Department (1997) *Who Decides? Making Decisions on Behalf of Mentally Incapacitated Adults*. A consultation paper. December 1997.

Montgomery J (1997) *Health Care Law*. New York: Oxford University Press.

Nelson JL and Nelson JL (1995) *The Patient in the Family: An Ethics of Medicine and Families*. London: Routledge.

Re C (1994) 1 All ER 819 (FD).

Re F (1989) 2 All ER 545.

Savulescu J and Momeyer RW (1997) Should informed consent be based on rational beliefs? *Journal of Medical Ethics* **23**: 282–288.

Schloendoff v. Society of New York Hospital (1914) 211 NY 125.

Sidaway v. Bethlem RHG (1985) All ER 643.

11

Embryos and Animals: Can We Justify Their Use in Research and Treatment?

Peter Singer

ABSTRACT

It is widely held that research on early human embryos is fraught with ethical problems, and either should not be done at all, or should be done only if, in some way, the embryos are not mere means to our ends. On the other hand, research on non-human animals is carried out on a vastly larger scale, and those who suggest that it should not be done at all, or that animals should not be used as mere means to our ends, are considered extremists. I suggest that the ethics of how we should treat a being depends, not on the species of the being, but on the being's level of awareness—and I consider the implications of this view for the ethics of research on human embryos and non-human animals.

INTRODUCTION

The following views about animals and embryos are widely held:

> Human embryos are early human beings and hence must be treated with the greatest respect. To use them for research or treatment intended to benefit others is to treat them as means to an end, and since it is always wrong to treat a human being as a means to an end, this cannot be justified.
>
> Animals are 'lower creatures' and, as such, are properly regarded as means to our ends. If our interests conflict with theirs, it is always their interests which have to give way. Hence the use of animals in research and treatment raises no ethical problems, unless the research is wantonly cruel (that is, causing pain or suffering when the results desired could be achieved without that pain and suffering).

I shall argue that these common attitudes are ethically indefensible. The attitudes we should hold are almost the mirror image of these two: whereas the use of embryos is relatively easy to justify, the use of animals is more difficult to defend.

The key to the attitudes we should have is the idea that ethics begins with a willingness to put ourselves in the position of the other, and ask whether we could defend an action, not only from our own perspectives, but if we had to live the lives of all those affected by it. (Hare, 1981). Suppose, for example, that we put ourselves in the situation of a prisoner of the Nazis, used in fatal decompression experiments. Clearly we could not defend a system that allows such experiments to be performed. The Nazi doctors themselves would never have performed them on their fellow 'Aryan' Germans. They were not putting themselves in the position of their victims, because they thought that their victims had, as 'non-Aryans', a morally inferior status. They could scarcely have denied that 'non-Aryans' suffer in very similar ways to 'Aryans' in such circumstances.

EMBRYOS

Consider now experiments on human embryos, involving the destruction of the embryo. We may say that, consistent with the principle I have outlined above, we must put ourselves in the position of the embryo in order to decide whether such experiments are justifiable. But when we put ourselves in the position of the embryo, what do we experience? Embryos do not have a brain or nervous system sufficiently developed for them to be capable of feeling pain (Burgess and Tawia, 1996; Derbyshire, 1999). It is safe to assume that they are not conscious, and have no feelings or experiences of any kind. So to put ourselves in their situation, even when they are being destroyed, is to experience nothing at all. We may as well put ourselves in the position of a lettuce being cut for a salad. (This essay discusses only research on the embryo *in vitro*, and such embryos have not, to date, ever developed for more than 2 weeks after fertilization.)

On this basis, other things being equal, there is nothing wrong with experimenting on human embryos. The qualification 'other things being equal' is intended to cover factors other than the destruction of the embryo in itself. For example, if the people from whom the gametes were obtained would be very upset to know that an embryo conceived from these gametes was used in experimentation, that would be a reason why it might be wrong to do so. The same would be true if the experiments were badly designed, and so used scarce research funds for no good purpose.

Some will protest that this is far too swift. If being non-conscious is sufficient reason for making it acceptable to carry out destructive experimentation on an embryo, why doesn't that apply to any one of us while we are asleep? And what about the potential of the embryo, which is entirely different from that of a lettuce?

The first question is easily answered. Although we are unconscious when we are asleep, we are conscious before we fall asleep, and our desires can reasonably be regarded as persisting, in a latent form, during sleep or other periods of temporary unconsciousness. We do not want to be killed while temporarily unconscious, so we can assume the same of others.

124

Ethical Dilemmas in Neurology

The question of potential requires a fuller answer. It is of course true that a human embryo could, given the right conditions, develop into a human being, whereas a lettuce will never develop into anything except a (flowering) lettuce. The question is whether this makes any difference to how we should treat the embryo before it has realized this potential. It could make a difference in various ways. For instance, since the embryo has the potential to become a person, it would be wrong to perform an experiment on it that had the consequence that, if the embryo does develop into a person, that person will suffer from an impairment. But this does not affect the ethics of experiments that result in the death of the embryo, rather than its impaired survival.

Another situation in which the potential of the embryo should make a difference is when we value the existence of the entity that the embryo has the potential to become. We might do so for various reasons. If the embryo has developed from the gametes of a childless couple on an in-vitro fertilization programme, they will want the embryo to develop into a child, and it would be wrong to use the embryo in a non-therapeutic experiment. Suppose, however, that the embryo is not wanted by the couple from whose gametes it developed. Let us assume that they have had other embryos fertilized, and as a result have had as many children as they wish to have. They are willing for this surplus embryo to be used for research. Should we, nevertheless, try to find couples who will carry this embryo to term, so that its potential can be realized? Why would we think that we ought to do that? Because we want there to be more people in the world? But if that is our goal, why are we so concerned about embryos, and not at all concerned about fertile couples who limit their families to one or two children when they could have half a dozen? If such couples are under no obligation to bring as many children as possible into the world—if we don't even see that as a good thing for them to do—then why does the fact that the embryo has the potential to develop into a person mean that there is any obligation on us to refrain from destroying it?

The remaining argument against embryo experimentation that we need to consider is that it is not so much the embryo's potential, as the fact that the embryo is already a living human being, and an innocent one, that makes it wrong to kill it. This argument parallels one we often hear in the context of the debate over abortion. The usual response from those seeking to defend abortion is to deny that the embryo, or fetus, is a living human being. I think this is tackling the argument at its strongest point. The embryo is a living human being. It is certainly alive, and it belongs to the species *Homo sapiens*, so what else can it be but human? It is also innocent of any wrongdoing. But does it follow from that that it is wrong to kill it? The argument:

> The embryo is an innocent living human being.
> Therefore it is wrong to kill the embryo.

is not a valid argument as it stands. It needs another premise:

> It is always wrong to kill an innocent human being.
> The embryo is an innocent living human being.
> Therefore it is wrong to kill the embryo.

This argument is valid. That means that if we accept its premises, we must also accept its conclusion. I have already said that I accept the second premise of the argument. It might be thought that the first premise is so obvious that we must accept it too. But that is not so. We must dare to ask: what is so special about being human that might make it always wrong to take innocent human life?

To help us think about this question, it is worth thinking about other innocent beings of whom we do not hold that it is always wrong to take their lives. For example, in most affluent societies people take the lives of cows, pigs and chickens simply because they like the taste of their flesh, even though they know that they could live just as long (perhaps longer) on a vegetarian diet. This seems to be a less serious reason for killing than the prospect of obtaining significant new information about the development of the embryo, yet people are much more concerned about killing embryos in the course of scientific research than they are about killing pigs because people like bacon. What could it be about human life that makes it so much more serious to kill any human being than to kill a pig?

If we search for capacities or qualities that make it more serious to kill a human being than a pig, we are likely to think first of those capacities that distinguish our own species from all others. A list of plausible candidates would include: self-awareness, reasoning, autonomy, the capacity to act morally, language, and the capacity to see oneself as existing over time, with a past and a future. These capacities all seem morally relevant, and distinctive of human beings. But there is an obvious problem. While they may be characteristics that normal humans beyond infancy have to a greater degree than any non-human animal, there are some humans who do not possess these characteristics to any degree, and others who do not possess them to a degree higher than that of, for example, pigs. Among those humans who do not possess these characteristics to any degree are anencephalics and embryos. Among those who do not possess them to a degree higher than a pig are all newborn and some severely intellectually disabled humans. So if it is not always wrong to take the life of an innocent pig, then these characteristics cannot justify the claim that it is always wrong to take the life of an innocent human being.

Nevertheless, human embryos and anencephalic infants are members of the species *Homo sapiens*. Is this not enough to justify the claim that it is always wrong to take their lives, when they are innocent of any wrongdoing? No, it is not. To regard species membership alone as sufficient to justify a higher moral status for a being is to take a moral stance that is logically parallel to racism and sexism. Speciesists, racists and sexists all say: the boundary of my own group is also the boundary of my concern. If you are a member of my group, you are superior to all those who are not members of my group. The speciesist favours a larger group than the racist, and so has a larger circle of concern; but all of these prejudices are equally wrong. They all use an arbitrary and morally irrelevant fact—membership of a race, sex or species—as if it were morally crucial.

Where does this leave us? It leaves us with the conclusion that, while human embryos are indeed innocent living human beings (in that they are innocent, alive, and members of the species *Homo sapiens*), this mere fact of species membership is not enough to make it wrong to kill them. We have found nothing to justify giving embryos a special status that makes it wrong to carry out destructive experiments on them. Therefore embryo experimentation is ethically acceptable as long as there is no objection from those who donated the gametes from which the embryo developed; there is no chance that the embryo will survive to become a damaged child; and the experiment is sufficiently well designed to be an effective use of the resources involved.

ANIMALS

If, as we saw earlier, putting ourselves in the position of others is fundamental to taking an ethical point of view, and if, as we have now seen, it is wrong to discriminate on the basis of species membership, then it seems clear that our readiness to put ourselves in the position of others must extend to all sentient beings affected by our actions, human and non-human. This means that the principle that should govern our relations with animals is the principle of equal consideration of interests. Essentially this means that if an animal feels pain, the pain matters as much as it does when a human feels pain—if the pains hurt just as much. *Pain is pain*, whatever the species of being that experiences it.

This does not, of course, mean that animals have the same rights as normal humans. It would be absurd to give animals the right to vote, but no more absurd than it would be to give that right to infants or to severely intellectually disabled human beings. Yet we still give equal consideration to the interests of humans in those categories. We do not raise them for food, or test new cosmetics in their eyes. Nor should we. But we do these things to non-human animals who are just as capable from suffering from it.

Animal experimentation starts from the idea that animals are ours to use, more or less as we please, as long as we avoid wanton cruelty. That is why for many years the standard way of assessing toxicity has been a test known as the LD_{50}. The name stands for lethal dose 50%. The object of the test is to find the dose level that will poison to death 50% of a sample of animals. Often more than one species of animal will be used. In the process of stepping up the dose until half the animals die, all of them will become very ill. They may suffer from nausea, diarrhoea, stomach cramps, thirst, and many other distressing symptoms. In this way, over the past two or three decades in Europe and North America, cruel, lingering deaths have been inflicted on tens of millions of sentient animals. Nor has this been done only to test potentially life-saving new drugs. The LD_{50} test has been routinely carried out on virtually every household product available in a supermarket or chemist shop, from food colourings and household cleaners to shaving cream, shampoos and cosmetics.

Now many government authorities no longer require the LD_{50}. That is a positive step, but until the animal liberation movement began to campaign against the LD_{50}, scientists had never spoken out against the unnecessary cruelty of the test. In any case, while the LD_{50} is not required, in most jurisdictions it is also not prohibited and in fact is still being carried out. Moreover, even when some slightly less cruel test is substituted for the classical LD_{50}, animals are still being poisoned, and still suffering, to test products that can only be described as totally unnecessary consumer trivia.

Product testing is only one example of the way in which we disregard the interests of laboratory animals. In schools of medicine and of the biological sciences, animals are given to students who are instructed to perform crude surgery, such as removing ovaries, to see how this affects their behaviour, when one film would teach just as much. No vital human benefits have resulted from such painful experimentation, and the major lesson students learn from the use of animals as tools for teaching is that their professors have no respect for sentient non-human animals.

As far as animal experimentation is concerned, the most important interests non-human animals have are the interests in not experiencing pain, fear, distress, and other forms of suffering; and in living conditions suited to their physical and psychological needs. These interests should be given the same weight as similar interests in humans. Doing so may not end all animal experimentation, but it would end the experimentation that does most to harm the interests that animals have.

It is arguable that some non-human animals do not have the same kind of interest in continued life that we do. Since we know that we exist over time, and are capable of forming desires not just for now, but also for tomorrow, next week, and next year, we have interests in continuing to live that are presumably beyond the comprehension of chickens, or mice (though there is evidence that chimpanzees, gorillas and orangutans are also self-aware). There is an ongoing debate about this issue which cannot be resolved here; it is enough to say that the principle of equal consideration may be compatible with the continuation of animal experimentation that kills animals, without inflicting pain or distress on them (Singer, 1993, Chs 4 & 5; 1995, Ch. 8).

It is a pity that, instead of responding positively to criticisms of animal experimentation, the medical research establishment in some countries, especially the United States, has waged a public relations war against the animal movement, designed to portray opponents of experiments on animals as 'terrorists' who base their appeal on emotions. Although some extremely unfortunate incidents have occurred, the handful of cases in which there have been injuries, or serious risk of injury to anyone, have been condemned by every major animal group, and by leading spokespeople for the animal movement. I have been speaking out against the use of violence by the movement for many years, and I repeated this plea in the Preface to the second edition of *Animal Liberation* (Singer, 1990). The overwhelming majority of the movement is concerned to prevent pain and suffering, wherever it occurs, and abhors violent attacks on experimenters, no matter how much suffering the experimenters may themselves have inflicted on animals.

It is also quite false to suggest that the animal liberation movement is based on an appeal to emotions. As I have indicated in this essay, the argument is an ethical one. People who are opposed to the exploitation of animals are no more 'animal lovers' than those who fought for civil rights for African Americans were 'nigger lovers'. Nor is the former more an emotional argument than the latter. Indeed, I doubt that any social movement has ever had as much input from reasoned argument by professional philosophers as the animal liberation movement. In that respect, far from being based on emotion, the animal liberation movement could be described as unique in the extent to which it is based on reasoning about an ethical issue.

If medical researchers are interested in defusing the controversy over animal experimentation, they are taking the wrong approach by going on the offensive in ways that do no credit to them. They would do much better to recognize that the use of animals in experimentation poses a serious ethical issue, and to work together with the animal movement to put their own house in order. This could begin by a joint attempt to eliminate experiments of the sort I have described above.

CONCLUSION

Most of the non-human animals used in research are clearly sentient beings, capable of feeling pain and other forms of distress. In contrast, no *in vitro* human embryos are capable of feeling pain, or anything else at all. Nor, subject to the consent of those from whom the gametes came, is there any reason why the potential of the embryo should affect the way in which we treat it, as long as it is not going to survive and develop into a conscious being. Hence, under these conditions, and other things being equal, the use of the human embryo in research is easier to justify than the use of the sentient animal.

REFERENCES

Burgess JA and Tawia SA (1996) When did you first begin to feel it?: locating the beginning of human consciousness. *Bioethics* **10**:1–26.
Derbyshire SWG (1999) Locating the beginnings of pain. *Bioethics* **13**:1–31.
Hare RM (1981) *Moral Thinking*. Oxford: Clarendon Press.
Singer P (1990) *Animal Liberation*, 2nd edn. New York: New York Review (first published 1975).
Singer P (1993) *Practical Ethics*, 2nd edn. Cambridge: Cambridge University Press (first published 1979).
Singer P (1995) *Rethinking Life and Death*. Oxford: Oxford University Press.

Funding and conflicts of interest

12

Does Private Practice Threaten Public Service or Enhance It?

Ian R Williams

ABSTRACT

Fifty years ago the National Health Service (NHS) was introduced in the United Kingdom. Despite imperfections it remains popular with the British public and is seen as an example of public service at its best. However, the underlying values of the NHS have been challenged by the continuing world-wide debate on health care reform. This essay looks at the legitimate concern which individuals have for the health of other members of their society and the way in which public service values and private practice influence both health and health care. It is argued that unequal access to health care, through the ability to pay, increases polarization in society and increases ill health. At the same time the availability and quality of health care available to the poorest, who have greatest need, is reduced. The effect on the individual, society, the medical profession and the NHS is detrimental. It is concluded that private practice damages public service.

INTRODUCTION

Neurology has changed dramatically over the last 20 years. Neurologists in the United Kingdom, once the ivory tower based thinkers, have discovered common disorders such as epilepsy and headache. New technology and new therapeutic agents have increased the range of diagnoses and possible interventions. The age of consumerism has nurtured a growth in public expectations. More is possible but much more is expected. With only one neurologist for every 200 000 people, demand exceeds supply. It would be interesting to ask whether the ivory towered origin was the reason for the relatively small number of neurologists in the United Kingdom; or indeed whether some kind of restrictive practice served, and continues to serve, the interests of the few. Whatever the answer to those questions there can be little doubt that, in times of shortage, people who wish to see a neurologist and have the means of achieving that goal will exercise their power. Those without power are without choice. Private practice is dependent on that polarization. Should neurologists respond to demand and provide a service for those powerful people—whatever the impact on those without power, and on society as a whole?

This is dangerous territory! To come to a conclusion, one way or the other, is to threaten cherished beliefs and livelihoods: even to raise the subject is to be seen to question the integrity and motives of physicians. Yet there can be few questions which so quickly lead to a discussion of the fundamentals of the form and function of health care and the role of the physician. In the present world-wide climate of health care reform, such a discussion assumes an even greater importance. Social, political and economic analysts are not reticent in proposing new roles, relationships and structures; unless doctors are also prepared to address the issue we will have to accept the outcome of their analysis. For the neurologist in the UK, the need to answer the question is perhaps even greater as the impact of the purchasing or commissioning arrangements in the NHS becomes clearer (Williams, 1992; Hopkins, 1994) and the debate about the organization of neurological services continues (Royal College of Physicians, 1996).

THE SERVICE

The funding and organization of health care has long been controversial. In the last 50 years advances in technology and changes in society have led both to increased demand and a reduced willingness to pay taxes. This has produced financial and other resource pressures which have uncovered ethical dilemmas which neither doctors nor politicians have found it easy to address. Is health care a service or a commodity? Should all citizens have a right to health care of the same standard, or of any standard, regardless of their ability to pay? Should clinicians have absolute freedom to prescribe whatever kind of treatment they wish even if its efficacy is not proven? Should patients have the right to choose whatever kind of treatment they wish even if its efficacy is not proven? What is the best way of organizing health care to make the best use of all available resources? As societies have struggled with these and other questions, the organization and provision of health care has changed. In the UK the health service reforms introduced a market of sorts and limited competition into the NHS. There was much talk of the privatization of health care and there has been a significant increase in the volume of private care (Calnan *et al.*, 1993). It is timely to ask whether there is good evidence that the existence of these two forms of health care side by side is injurious to the idea and practice of public service medicine and consequently to the health of the society.

The introduction of the NHS 50 years ago has been described as one of the great days in British history (Hennessy, 1993). The idea had taken 40 years to grow and 'at the time of its creation it was the first comprehensive system to be based not on the insurance principle ... but on the national provision of services available to everyone' (Klein, 1983). It was explicitly designed to improve the health of the public and to make a comprehensive range of health care available to all, regardless of ability to pay. Aneurin Bevan, whose political skills were largely responsible for winning the battle with a somewhat reluctant medical profession, stated that 'a free Health Service is a triumphant example of the superiority of collective action and public initiative applied to a segment of society where commercial principles are seen at their worst' (Bevan, 1952).

Bevan's analysis would not have come as a surprise to George Bernard Shaw who was in the main sympathetic to doctors, noting their relatively low income and the difficulties which their professional life entailed. He was, however, of the opinion that doctors were 'just like other Englishmen' and shared the many failings of human beings. In the preface to his play *'The Doctor's Dilemma'* he notes the many conflicts of interest between doctor and patient and between the wishes of the patient and the demands of society. He amusingly parodies the dilemma which he saw to be at the heart of private practice medicine. 'Could I not make better use of a pocketful of guineas than this man is making of his leg?' (Shaw, 1906). In his preface Shaw argues that the creation of a health service would be better for the patient, better for society, and better for the doctor. The Labour politicians elected in a landslide victory after the Second World War agreed with him and the great public service venture was begun.

Public service is based fundamentally on a recognition of the important role of society to provide a foundation for the life of the individual. It is thus in opposition to a view of society as purely a collection of individuals and sees freedom arising out of that sound basis of society rather than in the ability to have one's own needs satisfied whatever the effect on the needs of others. Plato noted that 'society originates, then ... because an individual is not self sufficient, but has many needs which he cannot supply himself' (Plato, c. 380 BC). He goes on to describe the demands that these needs place on the structure and organization of society and the expectations that members of society have of one another. His solution is not one that would necessarily find favour today! It is self evident that if individuals have an expectation that other citizens will play their part in maintaining a stable society, whether through growing food or manufacturing cars, it is important that they are fit and well enough to do so. It is also self evident that each individual within society will wish to be protected from contagious or infectious disease whether by vaccination, public health measures, or the prompt treatment of such diseases when they afflict other citizens. In discussing the reason for Bevan's commitment to the introduction of the NHS, Hennessy quotes Bevan as writing 'Society becomes more wholesome, more serene, and spiritually healthier if it knows that its citizens have at the back of their consciousness the knowledge that not only themselves, but all their fellows, have access, when ill, to the best that medical skill can provide' (Hennessy, 1993). The NHS, as an outstanding example of public service, was created to bring about improvements in society as well as in the health of the individual. In asking whether private practice has an influence on public service it is, therefore, necessary to examine its impact on the individual patient, on the NHS and society as a whole, and on the practice of medicine.

For each individual the NHS provides the full range of care which is, with a few exceptions, free of charge at the point of use. Most needs are met in primary care where access to the general practitioner (GP) is easy and rapid and a wide range of investigation and treatment can be undertaken. There is little private practice undertaken at this level. However, if referral for more specialist care is required the situation is somewhat different: a very significant proportion of elective surgery is undertaken in the private sector. In 1989, 13% of the UK population was covered by some form of health insurance (Calnan *et al.*, 1993) and 30% of hip replacements were done privately in 1991–1992 (Yates, 1995). The long waiting time for appointments to see the specialist is one obvious reason for people to make this choice. In a detailed survey of waiting times in the NHS and private sectors, Yates (1995) found large differences: in the private sector the average wait for an orthopaedic consultation was 2 weeks while the same person would have had to wait 25 weeks in the NHS. The same is true for admission to hospital. The median waiting time for elective admission was 42 days in the NHS compared to 9 days in private beds within NHS hospitals in 1994–95 (Williams, 1997). While the difference was greatest for procedures such as inguinal hernia or cataract, the wait was about twice as long for NHS patients awaiting breast excision or coronary artery grafting as for their private practice counterparts. In these circumstances there is clearly something to be gained by buying private care if it can be afforded. Waiting times were, however, not the only factor to determine use of the private sector in the study of Calnan *et al.* (1993). Choice of time, and to a lesser extent of consultant, figured, as did the social status conferred by being a private patient.

It would appear to be all gain for the individual patient, although in choosing a private hospital for their treatment patients may not realize the extent to which modern medicine is a team effort; they may also not be aware of the limited support available in many private hospitals in the UK from resident medical staff or on-site colleagues should anything go wrong (Currie, 1996). It is also possible that investigations and procedures which would in other situations be felt to be unnecessary are performed in order to secure the fee. While it is difficult to interpret the figures, the disproportion between the percentage of the population insured and the number of procedures performed in the private sector suggests either that those who cannot afford private treatment are being under-treated or those paying for care are being over-treated. George Bernard Shaw would have had no doubt which was true (Shaw, 1906). The benefits may not be quite what they appear. Caveat emptor!

THE CONSULTANT

Does the choice of one individual to use private care influence the health of other individuals? Sadly, in a situation where consultants are able to work both in the NHS and in the private sector the answer has to be yes. Doctors cannot be in two places at once: while they are treating the private patient they cannot be treating the NHS patient. In a society where the private patient and the NHS patient were equivalent the choice would be less important. It could even be argued that by seeing some people outside the NHS the pressure on waiting list and clinic time is reduced. However, not only do consultants tend to see more patients in a given time in the NHS than in private practice, but the selection of patients who can afford to pay, ahead of those who cannot, is probably the reverse of what is needed. There is ample evidence to show that socio-economic standing correlates well with health (Black *et al.* 1992) and that people with a higher income spend more on health care (Pauly, 1992). Thus the choice of the more affluent to be seen earlier and at greater length displaces poorer and possibly more needy people further down the waiting list where they may be seen by junior staff or given a shorter consultation with a consultant. This undesired and undesirable effect on the public service could only be removed if consultants were employed only in one or other sector.

During the negotiations which led to the creation of the NHS the medical profession was not wholly supportive. Among the concessions needed to convince the consultants that they should take part was the agreement that they should be able to continue their private practice alongside the NHS work. This led to the adoption of a contract of employment which was, and remains, impossible to understand or enforce. The maximum part time contract allowed consultants to give up about 10% of their salary in return for the opportunity to earn an unrestricted amount in private practice. The contract stated that such consultants would be expected to devote 'substantially the whole of their time' to the NHS. Many of those engaged in private practice would argue that this means that they work harder than full-time NHS colleagues, fulfilling the terms of their agreement with the NHS and undertaking private practice in addition. Whatever the truth of this, the NHS employs the most expensive part of its workforce on the basis of an uninterpretable contract as a result of the need to ensure the continuation of private practice medicine! It is hard to know whether any other course was open to Bevan and his colleagues but it is a legacy which continues to threaten the public service in a variety of ways.

The inability to be precise about what can be expected of consultants makes conversations about workload difficult. Yates (1995) went to extraordinary lengths to try to establish the job content of the surgeons he studied. Average operating times for each surgeon in the NHS were low and there was a considerable commitment to private practice during normal working hours. With long waiting lists to see consultants in the NHS and then long waits for admission to the ward for treatment it would almost certainly be in the public interest to ensure that each surgeon performed more operations for the NHS each week and spent less time in his private practice. With a more practical contract of employment the NHS could bring this about. Whatever the resulting impact on health care there can be little doubt that the contract makes management in the NHS much more difficult.

Another area of managerial difficulty arises because of the lack of information on consultant activity. From publicly available figures for the NHS it is impossible to know whether procedures are performed by a consultant or his junior staff: there are no figures for private practice. Yates unearthed several examples which showed a lamentably low NHS activity by consultants who were busy in private practice. His report was suppressed because his 'comments on private practice were too strong' (Yates, 1995). Suppression of such comments and research is certainly not good for the public service.

There is a wealth of rumour and anecdote about the length of the waiting list to see specialists who also engage in private practice. It is suggested that long waiting lists increase the number of private referrals and that it is therefore in the specialist's interest to keep his NHS waiting list long (Light, 1997). Although the coincidence of long waiting lists with high private referral rates is a generally observed phenomenon, it is at least as likely that the list is long in spite of the efforts of the specialist to contain it. In these circumstances, however, the specialist finds the atmosphere and pace in his private practice much preferable to the frenzy and dissatisfaction in the overloaded NHS clinic. Whether it can be seen as damaging to the public service that the specialist has an alternative in such situations is far from clear: it is certainly not proven. More damaging is the situation which has arisen in some localities since the creation of the internal market in the NHS. When access to a specialist clinic in the NHS becomes difficult, because of a long waiting list, the GP fundholder is free to buy the time of that same overpressed specialist to have his own patients seen ahead of the queue. Thus the specialist has even less time for the NHS patients and takes income away from the hospital. There can be few employers who allow their employees to set up in direct competition and allow them to control the process which feeds their business. While some may feel that competition is good for quality and access it surely damages the NHS when it is powerless to make the decisions necessary to improve care. Neurology is certainly not immune to this contagion!

SOCIETY

It is not only in the NHS that patients suffer because of physicians' choices. Iglehart (1993), studying Medicaid in the US, quotes studies which show that it is difficult to get physicians to take part in the Medicaid programme, partly because of inadequate payment. Only one-third of practising physicians participate fully in the programme. Mullan notes that inner city hospitals in the US have to depend on foreign graduates because of the long-standing tradition of using medical trainees in institutions which serve the indigent (Mullan, 1997). It appears that the ability to provide care for those who need it most is compromised by the ability of physicians to earn more by looking after the more affluent, both in the US and the UK. In both situations it would be hard to say that private practice enhanced public service.

Less obvious, but probably still important, is the effect that the existence and use of private practice have on society. In his book *Choose Freedom*, which examines the future of democratic socialism, Roy Hattersley lists the effects of a private sector in health. He states that it exemplifies and perpetuates division in society: 'it does more than offer the recipients of private provision a superior service. It depresses the service provided in the public sector'. He further comments that it isolates the influential from the failings of the public service and makes it less likely that they will be corrected. 'The abolition of private medicine and education would, by any sensible analysis, increase the sum of liberties' (Hattersley, 1987). As a previous deputy leader of the UK Labour party his views are perhaps not surprising: that does not mean that they are wrong! There is now an increasing body of work which looks beyond the longstanding observation that poverty and ill health are linked, to examine the effects of differences within society. Wilkinson reviews some of the evidence that shows that more egalitarian societies are more cohesive and that better integration into a network of social relations benefits health (Wilkinson, 1997). Thus it may be supposed that those things which promote or proclaim inequality also promote ill health in society. At first sight this would appear only to affect the excluded and deprived people, but, in concluding, Wilkinson notes that with rising crime, drug misuse and poor educational performance the rest of society cannot long remain insulated from the effects of high levels of relative deprivation.

CONCLUSION

The majority of this essay has been concerned with the situation in the UK where the same individual can work both in the NHS and in private practice, but what little evidence I have quoted from the US points in the same direction. Although I would like to be charitable I can find little evidence to support the contention that private practice enhances public service. From the effect on the drawing up of the consultant contract at the beginning of the NHS, to the ability of consultants to divert resources from the NHS, private practice has impaired the ability of the public service to deliver. Furthermore it has probably contributed to increased division in society, taken skilled care from those who have greatest need in order to provide for those with least need, and in both these ways has allowed a greater amount of ill health and suffering than would otherwise have been the case. Whatever the commitment of those many hard working and compassionate individuals within the NHS who also work in the private sector, the net effect of their contribution is damaging to the public good. Private practice, which is concerned with maximizing the benefit to the individual, is in conflict with public service, which serves the public good.

REFERENCES

Bevan A (1952) *In Place of Fear*, p. 85. London: Heinemann.

Black D *et al.* (1992) The Black Report. In: *Inequalities in Health*, 2nd edn (eds P Townsend and N Davidson). London: Penguin.

Calnan M, Cant S and Gabe J (1993) *Going Private. Why People Pay for their Health Care*. Buckingham: Open University Press.

Currie D (1996) BUPA subscription? That will do nicely. *British Medical Journal* **313**:431.

Hattersley R (1987) *Choose Freedom. The Future for Democratic Socialism*, pp. 145–147. London: Penguin.

Hennessy P (1993) *Never Again. Britain 1945–1951*. London: Vintage.

Hopkins A (1994) Economic change and health service reforms: likely impact on teaching, practice, and research in neurology. *Journal of Neurology, Neurosurgery and Psychiatry* **57**:667–671.

Iglehart JK (1993) The American Health Care System. Medicaid. *New England Journal of Medicine* **336**:1601–1603.

Klein R (1983) *The Politics of the National Health Service*, p. 1. London: Longman.

Light DW (1997) The real ethics of rationing. *British Medical Journal* **315**:112–115.

Mullan F (1997) The National Health Service Corps and Inner-City Hospitals. *New England Journal of Medicine* **336**:1601–1603.

Pauly MV (1992) Fairness and Feasibility in National Health Care Systems. *Health Economics* **1**:896–900.

Plato (*c.*380 BC) The republic. In: *The Republic* (trans HDP Lee) (1955), p. 102. Harmondsworth: Penguin.

Royal College of Physicians (1996) *The District General Hospital as a Resource for the Provision of Neurological Services*. London: Royal College of Physicians of London.

Shaw GB (1906) The doctor's dilemma. In: *Prefaces by Bernard Shaw* (1938) p. 237. London: Odhams.

Wilkinson RG (1997) Socioeconomic determinants of health. Health inequalities: relative or absolute material standards? *British Medical Journal* **314**:591–595.

Williams B (1997) Utilisation of National Health Service hospitals in England by private patients 1989–95. *Health Trends* **29**:21–25.

Williams IR (1992) Neurology in the market place. *Journal of Neurology, Neurosurgery and Psychiatry* **55** (Suppl):15–18.

Yates J (1995) *Private Eye, Heart and Hip. Surgical Consultants, the National Health Service and Private Medicine*. Edinburgh: Churchill Livingstone.

13

The Gulf War Syndrome and the Military Medic: Whose Agent is the Physician?

Edmund G Howe

ABSTRACT

This essay discusses three ethical conflicts which arose for military physicians during and after the Gulf War. All involve the conflict between serving their patients and serving the military. Initially, background material is provided, such as analyses of the principle of military medical triage and of military physicians' role-specific ethic. Then the specific conflicts are discussed: whether military physicians should have forced servicepersons to take protective agents, when the military should have informed servicepersons that they may have been exposed to toxic chemicals, and whether military doctors should tell the truth about the possible psychogenic or physical causation of the Gulf War Syndrome. Recommendations are given regarding what military physicians should do in each of these instances.

INTRODUCTION

Ethical dilemas arise for all physicians when they face conflicting obligations. Such conflicts occur, for example, when doctors must give priority to the public health over that of individual patients, and when psychiatrists see patients who may harm a third party. It occurred most recently and notoriously when some managed care organizations required doctors not to inform patients about treatments that these organizations did not offer. This was the so-called 'gag rule'.

In the practice of military medicine, the ethical aspects of these conflicts are essentially similar, but the stakes are much higher. If, for instance, the military endeavour does not prevail, as the Second World War particularly illustrates, the outcome may include such heinous acts as genocide. As another example, some individual servicepersons have access to incredibly destructive weaponry. Thus, if they acquire serious emotional difficulties, this could result in their inflicting exceptional harm.

139

These much greater stakes mean that it is important to determine, what, if anything, military physicians should do differently from their civilian colleagues when they encounter such dilemas. This chapter will discuss this question using three examples which involve the Gulf War. The first two arose during combat: whether servicepersons should have been forced to take protective agents against biological and chemical warfare; and whether they should have been informed that they may have been exposed to toxic chemicals after coalition forces blew up an ammunitions dump in Iraq and, if they should have been told, when.

The third dilemma continues to confront physicians today: how to treat servicepersons with the Gulf War Syndrome. This dilemma is similar to one which civilian doctors face routinely when they treat patients with symptoms which may be wholly or partly psychogenic—namely, the degree to which they should be honest with these patients regarding their symptoms' origin. The question is also discussed in Essay 2 of this book.

This essay initially describes some differences in the practice of military medicine, because I believe that the nature of these differences must be understood to appreciate the dilemmas which arose in the Gulf and their resolutions. It then describes the dilemmas enumerated above that arose there. Finally, in discussing problems when treating patients with the Gulf War Syndrome, it presents what I believe to be the optimal approach at the present time. I suggest that the model careproviders should use is based on one that some neurologists now use when treating patients with psychogenic seizures.

These topics are discussed under these subheadings: basic differences; dilemmas in the Gulf; Gulf War Syndrome; and analogies with other 'possibly psychosomatic' disorders. The essay concludes by defending the view that, notwithstanding the generally greater stakes in the military, in most instances, it is ethically possible and preferable to give priority to deontological values, such as truth-telling, as is the case in civilian medicine.

BASIC DIFFERENCES

The values prioritized by military physicians during combat are in some instances the opposite of those prioritized in civilian practice. For instance, during battle, when many servicepersons have been injured, military physicians may treat less severely injured servicepersons first so that these servicepersons can continue to fight, even though, as a result of this practice, severely injured servicepersons who could have been saved may die. This practice is uncommon, but it does occur. The best known instance in which this occurred was during the Second World War. Since penicillin had only then first become available, supplies were limited. Military doctors gave penicillin to servicepersons with venereal disease so that they could return to battle, even though, as a result, others with life-threatening infections died (Beecher, 1970).

Civilian careproviders, in contrast, would probably have given priority in this situation to saving patients' lives.

The discrepant priority adopted in this situation is referred to as 'military medical triage'. It primarily has two ethical justifications. First, society's decision that war is necessary is presumed to be ethically valid. Second, it may be justified in terms of maintaining equity among service personnel.

The first justification involves considerations about what constitutes a just war. These considerations go beyond the scope of this essay; nonetheless, brief comment is necessary. Just war theory must be considered in this context in its widest sense. That is, considerations should include not only whether the war is just but whether the means of warfare used are justifiable. Since the Second World War involved the prevention of genocide, as alluded to already, it is paradigmatic of a war which was justifiable. It would, in fact, have been immoral not to fight this war. The use of the atom bomb to end the war, is, in contrast, open to question since it involved the death of numerous civilians.

Presuming, then, that a war and its means are just, military physicians are deemed justified in not helping ill or injured servicepersons. They may be obligated to give priority to the military medical triage principle if this is considered necessary to win the war. This necessity is, however, to be determined by military officers presumed to have the greatest knowledge and expertise in this area, not physicians.

The implications for military physicians are profound. Military physicians must agree when they join the military to subordinate and sacrifice the priorities they would hold as civilian physicians. They implicitly promise to abide by the decisions of military officers of higher rank.

Military physicians agreeing to accept this moral priority are adopting what is referred to as a role-specific ethic. This means that they subscribe to the moral requirements of that role: this includes accepting their superior officers' judgements as opposed to exercising their own discretion and making ethical judgements themselves. However, a most difficult quandary can still arise for military physicians: when, if ever, should they violate this role-specific ethic and exercise independent judgement? The military itself requires them, as all servicepersons, to disobey an order which is illegal or unethical. The difficulty, of course, is deciding when this is the case.

An example in which this dilemma arose occurred during the Second World War. In the South Pacific, commanding officers decided that even servicepersons with severe malaria and dysentery should return to the front. According to their role-specific ethic, military physicians could have stated their objections but, if they were overruled, would have been expected to comply. Some believe that under these circumstances they should have objected. General Stelling stated, for instance, that he believes that military physicians should have insisted on the evacuation of these servicepersons and that it was 'a disgrace' that they did not (Hopkins *et al.*, 1969). Even these physicians may, however, have been unaware of critical considerations known to their commanding officers. Their commanders may have known, for example, that without these extra servicepersons enemy forces could imminently prevail but that large numbers of reinforcement troops could reverse that if they were already on their way.

Thus, if military physicians violate their role-specific ethic and insist on the evacuation of servicepersons such as these, because they are ill, they would fulfill their medical obligation to individual servicepersons who are their patients, but would violate mutually exclusive obligations to the military and to other servicepersons. That is, they would violate the explicit promise they gave to the military to follow orders when joining. They would also violate an implicit promise they also make to all servicepersons at this time—to serve the miltary's goals so that both the military mission can be accomplished and the greatest numbers of servicepersons can come out of battle alive.

Second, the practice of military medical triage is ethically justified on the ground that it maintains equity among all servicepersons, whether they have been injured or continue to fight at the front. The lives of servicepersons at the front are, of course, always at risk. When military physicians treat first servicepersons who are injured but can return to the front as opposed to those closer to death and severely injured, as stated, this may result in the death of those more severely injured. For both those who return to battle and those who remain too injured to return, the risk of death remains.

Civilian physicians, in contrast, treat first those patients who have the greatest risk of dying. They may depart from this practice when mass casualties occur during natural disasters, such as earthquakes or floods, so that the greatest number of patients can survive, but, since there is no military mission, they will never allow some patients to die for the sake of the mission.

A subgroup of servicepersons whose individual interests also may be sacrificed for those of society is servicepersons with combat fatigue (Veatch, 1977). These servicepersons find themselves overwhelmed by the stress of combat and become unable to function on the battlefield. Military psychiatrists customarily treat these patients with food, brief rest, and the expectation that they will return to duty quickly. Most respond to this expectation and return to duty after just a few days.

A justification military physicians have for following this practice is that, if military physicians do not act in this manner, innumerable additional servicepersons, for unconscious or conscious reasons, could also develop combat fatigue (Howe, 1986). This could occur because their symptoms would enable them to gain exit from the battlefield, and thus they could avoid further combat and the great risk it poses of death. Civilian doctors, in contrast, might encourage patients overwhelmed by stress to avoid any further exposure to it. It is also believed on the basis of military psychiatrists' and servicepersons' past experience, that if servicepersons suffering from combat fatigue return to battle, so long as they survive it, they are likely to be emotionally much better off. It is believed that if they are relieved from front line duty permanently they become exceptionally vulnerable to experiencing exorbitant guilt because other members of their unit may die when they will have survived (Howe, 1986).

DILEMMAS IN THE GULF

PROTECTIVE AGENTS

The first ethical conflict which arose in the Persian Gulf War was whether to require servicepersons to take a vaccine against botulism and a drug, pyridostigmine, to protect them from biological and chemical warfare, respectively (Howe and Martin, 1991).

These agents had not been fully tested for these specific purposes. They had been found in other, limited contexts to be safe and efficacious, but it would have been unethical to expose humans as research subjects to these vaccines and this weaponry to determine the extent to which, according to the usual standards of scientific certainty, these agents were safe and efficacious. This use of these agents to protect servicepersons had nothing to do with the usual purposes of research. Sources of military intelligence had indicated that Iraq possessed biological weaponry such as botulism and chemical weapons. It was known that both are highly deadly. Subsequent findings have shown that this intelligence was correct.

Iraq may have avoided using this weaponry only because Saddam Hussein believed that the US would retaliate with nuclear weaponry. Whether this would have occurred is open to speculation.

Yet whether or not this was a false belief, and whether the US purposefully acted to convey it, are related at least in theory to military physicians' obligation to give priority to their duties to the military. That is, as previously indicated, military physicians giving priority to military needs is justifiable only if two prior conditions have been met: the reasons for going to war are just, and the means by which the war is being waged are just.

These determinations are more equivocal than may appear. Questions remaining unanswered in regard to the Gulf War, for example, are whether the US should have applied other non-violent sanctions longer before going to war, and when war efforts should have stopped once it was known that Iraq was defeated. Similarly, suppose that the US had determined that even if Iraq did use biological or chemical weapons, the US would not have responded with nuclear attack. If, not withstanding this determination, the US indicated it would use nuclear weaponry. This would be purposeful deceit. If this deceit was deemed an unjust means of waging war, military physicians giving priority to their military obligations might be unjustifiable as well.

It was decided that servicepersons should be required to take these protective agents for the following reasons. If Iraq used this weaponry, servicepersons who did not take the vaccine would die, and other servicepersons left without these servicepersons' help or trying to save them also might die. The success of the war effort might itself have been placed in jeopardy. Then, of course, even if the US had previously decided not to use nuclear weaponry, it might have had to reconsider this decision.

The use of such agents without servicepersons' consent had been challenged in court prior to the time the need to give these agents arose. The court ruled that the military could give these protective agents to servicepersons without their consent (Doe v. Sullivan, 1991). The rationales for this decision were consistent with the principles of military medical triage aforementioned. This use was deemed necessary to benefit the greatest number of servicepersons by saving their lives, and, in doing so, to further the likelihood of the military's winning the war.

After it was decided that the military could require servicepersons to use these protective agents, the amount of vaccine initially available was not enough to protect all servicepersons. This resulted in three ethical problems.

The first problem was who should receive the limited vaccine that was available. The principle of military medical triage dictated that it should be given to those servicepersons whose protection was most necessary for the military's success.

To meet the military's needs maximally, it might be justifiable to give priority to saving the lives of those in command, those who could save more servicepersons' lives by providing medical care, or those more critical to the survival of others in some other way. Among the more difficult of these determinations was whether the limited amounts of vaccine should be given to servicepersons at the front or at the rear.

The second problem was the extent to which military physicians should tell those servicepersons not offered the vaccine that it was being given to other servicepersons, and whether they should tell servicepersons receiving the vaccine that one dose was insufficient to protect them fully. The consideration principally at stake here was the induction of fear. If servicepersons panicked because they were unprotected or inadequately protected, large numbers of servicepersons, due to fear, could become immobilized. This concern was analogous, then, to the concern about 'opening the floodgates' when servicepersons have combat fatigue, as considered above. Servicepersons, in general, were informed; some were upset, but there was no widespread panic.

This outcome illustrates a psychological phenomenon which may explain some of the rage experienced by servicepersons in response to not being told that they may have been exposed to toxic chemicals in the Gulf, the next issue that I shall consider. This phenomenon potentially is immensely important to both policy makers and clinicians: that is, if persons are told the truth and what to expect, even if the truth is frightening, they may be much better able to handle their fear well. This possibility extends even to information which is uncertain. If persons are informed that an outcome is uncertain, they may cope much better than if they are not informed at all. This may be because, if information is disclosed, it implies that its consequences can be borne or at least those with information can be trusted, whereas, if information is not disclosed, it may imply that its implications are so overwhelming that the information cannot be disclosed and/or that grounds for trust are absent. For both these reasons, then, withholding information that an event may be catastrophic may make a catastrophic outcome a self-fulfilling prophecy.

This psychological possibility is illustrated by patients' response after the subway sarin gas attack in Tokyo, Japan, in 1995 (Komai, 1995). Twelve persons died, 5050 were injured. Patients presenting to hospitals were fully informed about what was and what was not known. St. Luke's International Hospital, to which 610 patients came, informed them immediately that they might encounter 'terrible mental shock'. As this makes clear, they were given the worst possibility they could expect. It may be that, in large part, as a result of their receiving this information, the psychiatric sequelae these patients experienced were minimal (Komai, 1998).

The third problem encountered in the Gulf was whether military physicians should require the servicepersons designated as most in need of the protective vaccine for the success of the mission to take it, or it go only to those servicepersons who wanted it. There were two reasons for those in authority in the Gulf to make this decision on the spot, in spite of their superior authorities' decision, after long deliberation in the States, that these servicepersons should be required to take these agents even without their consent. First, they had access to the most up-to-date information, such as whether Iraq actually would use this weaponry. Second, they could best take into account, based on what they saw before them, how the servicepersons in the combat theatre actually would react.

Medical authorities in the Gulf advised their superiors to allow local commanders to use their discretion. These commanders could then allow servicepersons individually to choose whether or not to take the vaccine. In making this recommendation, the medical authorities exercised independent discretion. Yet their recommendation, as stated, contradicted a policy which had been determined after long deliberation and which, indeed, after the court's decision, was sanctioned by law. In going against this 'wisdom of their superiors', they took a risk. Like Stelling, they risked responding to seemingly important but short-sighted exigencies. Retrospectively, this independent judgement may have seemed imprudent, such that these medical authorities would have been better off not second guessing those who had decided otherwise, originally, back in Washington.

The dilemma faced by the medical authorities in the Gulf is common to servicepersons in other contexts and stems from the existence of both a formal and an informal role-specific ethic, which may contradict each other. That is on the 'formal' level, these physicians were expected to make an on-the-spot decision independently. This is what they knew explicitly they were permitted and encouraged to do. On another 'informal' level, they were expected to defer to others who had decided this issue before it devolved to them. Implicitly, they knew, then, that if they used their independent judgement and made different decisions from their superiors, and if retrospectively, these judgements were poor ones, in informal ways, as in career advancement, they could be held accountable.

To illustrate how these two levels of a role-specific ethic operate in another context, servicepersons are explicitly encouraged and expected to disobey orders if the orders are illegal or immoral. If, however, they refuse to obey an order because they believe that it is illegal or immoral, they do so at their peril. In this case the potential adverse sanctions are greater: if the order is, in fact, subsequently deemed legal and moral, they can be court-martialled for refusing to obey an order.

Since those who refuse on these grounds risk courts-martial, this illustrates that they are also expected to comply with the decisions of their superiors if they are in doubt. Thus, they can face mutually exclusive, contradictory expections. Simply stated, their more formal expectation or role-specific ethic requires military physicians—as all servicepersons—to exercise independent judgment. Their more informal expectation or role-specific ethic makes it strongly in their interest to defer their judgement to their superiors if they have doubt.

Since these formal and informal role-specific ethics conflict, military physicians and other servicepersons making independent judgements may experience more difficulty and, accordingly, require more courage than is initially apparent. This conflict and the resultant need for courage illustrated, also, in the following two examples.

During the Vietnam conflict, for the US, the Geneva Convention of 1949 was in effect. Military physicians had an obligation under this international law to treat captured enemy servicepersons in a manner equal to their own, but not to treat injured civilians equally (Howe, 1997). What should a military physician have done, then, when a civilian's need for treatment was substantially greater than that of a serviceperson? One physician describes what occurred as follows: 'Triage had a wall to wall carpet of wounded bodies with doctors and corpsmen skipping over, between and around them: kneeling, sitting and standing, but never stopping … "leave those damn civilians alone; there are dying marines all around you. I'll court martial the next one who touches a wounded civilian"' (Parrish, 1962). This order was legal. Was it unethical? Should military physicians have used their independent judgement and violated it? In this case, since these physicians had an order, they faced two expectations or role-specific ethics which contradicted one another. Formally and explicitly, they were expected to obey an order, and to disobey an order if the order was illegal or immoral. Informally and implicitly, however, they knew that if they were in doubt regarding the immorality of this order, to best protect their own interests, they should comply. Military physicians exercising their independent judgement and treating civilians in this situation would have required exceptional courage.

This situation can be usefully contrasted with a superior officer's ordering military physicians to treat their own servicepersons before treating captured enemy servicepersons who are worse off. Many military physicians serving in the Persian Gulf in fact believed that, morally, under these circumstances, they should treat their own servicepersons first (Carter, 1994). Legally, in this instance, they must do otherwise. Military physicians are obligated under international law to treat enemy servicepersons equally, and under military law to uphold international law. In this instance, they have no role-specific ethic to withhold this treatment. Consequently, military physicians who believe they should not treat enemy servicepersons in this situation are mistaken.

The medical officers in the Gulf who exercised independent judgement showed courage, then, but why did they depart from the previous judgement and make the decision they did? Perhaps for only the reasons given above. Yet civilian physicians place a high priority on requiring informed consent; this also may have influenced the decision.

The military is increasingly under the scrutiny of the greater society and accordingly is under more pressure to adhere to civilian standards except in those instances in which a convincing case can be made that it should not. Several recent examples support this. The best example, perhaps, is the recent alteration to military policy in regard to servicepersons who are homosexual (Jones and Koshes, 1995). Another is the new emphasis on providing treatment to servicepersons who have problems with substance abuse (Kallen *et al.*, 1989).

Is this trend desirable? The horrors of war are many. It may seem unequivocal that, to reduce these horrors, the military should follow civilian standards wherever possible and when the military believes that its standard of practice should be different, the military should have the burden of making this case. But who will judge whether or not military authorities have met this burden and shown that the standard of practice in the military should be different? Those who would judge whether the military has made this case may, somewhat like Stelling, not be sufficiently informed regarding military exigencies to assess their priorities validly.

Some in the civilian population may, in addition, project negative feelings they hold toward the military when they make these judgements. This prejudice may make it impossible to find a group which is both representative of the population and sufficiently unbiased to make these judgements objectively.

Some argue, based on the considerations just stated, that the military made a mistake when it sought permission from a civilian court to use these prophylactic agents without servicepersons' consent in the Gulf. Rather, they argue, it should have used its own discretion. Otherwise, they contend, if civilians had decided they should not give the military this permission and Iraq had then used this weaponry, inordinate numbers of servicepersons now would be dead.

POTENTIAL EXPOSURE

In late January and February 1991, coalition forces blew up chemical munition sites in central Iraq. One of these sites released mustard gas and the chemical sarin, the poison used in the Tokyo subway system (Roberts, 1996). When it first became clear that this had occurred, a number of questions arose.

It was unknown how many servicepersons might have been exposed to the effects of these chemicals and, if they were exposed, what, if any, the effects could be. One possible response was to disclose all information regarding this event immediately, regardless of what the consequences might be. Another response was to study the situation first to attempt to discern the possible effects prior to divulging that these events had occurred.

If this information had been disclosed at once, adverse consequences for individuals and the military could have occurred. Servicepersons could have panicked and, falsely believing they were exposed, developed psychogenic symptoms in response to having received this information (Haberman, 1987). Further, when persons have somatic symptoms caused or exacerbated by psychological factors, such as stress, if they have reason to believe that these symptoms are caused by physical factors, these symptoms may, it is believed, be more likely to become entrenched. This may particularly be likely if, in addition, there is a possibility of financial reward, as from a suit, or of some other kind of secondary gain (Binder and Rohling, 1996).

After a year-long study the Senate Veterans Affairs Committee faulted the Pentagon for denying any exposure for five years and then releasing an estimate of the number of servicepersons exposed which was 'far too high' because it was based on a 'computer model that was "fundamentally flawed".' and failing to recreate the weapons bunker and atmospheric conditions which existed at that time accurately. The committee concluded that the result did 'more to confuse and alarm Gulf War veterans, both those healthy and ill, than to help them' (McAllister, 1998).

Different values favour different actions. The principle of respect for persons requires that this information should have been disclosed to servicepersons at once. Yet paternalistic concerns support greater caution. Disclosing this information initially could have had adverse repercussions on both servicepersons and the military. It could have created psychologically caused emotional and physical symptoms among servicepersons only possibly exposed. And if servicepersons who may have been exposed became symptomatic and unable to function as a result of having learned this information, they could have become unable to serve effectively in the military. The loss of these servicepersons would reduce the effectiveness of the mission.

Information was not immediately disclosed, and, as further study ensued, this decision seemed more and more ethically problematic.

> In June, after four years of maintaining that gulf soldiers were not exposed to any chemical or biological weapons, the Pentagon acknowledged that up to 400 Army personnel could have come in contact with poison gas. That number quickly rose to 5,000 and, earlier this month, to more than 15,000 [service personnel] who were within a 50-kilometer (31-mile) circle of Kamisiyah. (McAllister, 1996)

Yet the more general question this incident posed remains. What if, for example, initial data on a few patients suggested the possibility that the Gulf War Syndrome was caused by an HIV-like virus activated by stress? Patients with this virus could infect loved ones. This information would be highly preliminary and its significance unknown. Should it be made public, immediately, regardless? An inextricably related question, of course, is who should decide.

GULF WAR SYNDROME

When servicepersons began to present with symptoms which came to be known as the Gulf War Syndrome, some believed that the protective agents had caused it. Coker, reviewing the British experience, for example, hypothesized that 'the ever present threat of biological and chemical attack, with the need to get in and out of Individual Protective Equipment, with the resulting physiological degradation, must have imposed constant physical and mental stress on personnel', and that the smoke from oil-well fires and a host of agents in combination with pyridostigmine bromide 'might have given rise to neurotoxic effects' (Coker, 1996).

Others believed that the toxic chemicals released from the blown-up ammunition dumps caused these symptoms. Eddington and Zaid reported, for example, that low-level chemical exposure, such as the exposure servicepersons in the vicinity would have undergone, had been shown to cause motor skill deficits and cognitive problems in primates (Eddington and Zaid, 1997).

A Presidential Advisory Committee tasked with reviewing all the evidence concluded that exposure had, indeed, occurred, but that this did not imply 'long-term health effects in those exposed' (Presidential Advisory Committee, 1996). The Senate Veterans Affairs Committee mentioned earlier, which has been highly critical of the military for failing to keep accurate records, simply concluded, 'There is insufficient evidence at this time to prove or disprove that there was actual low-level exposure of any troops to chemical weapon nerve agents or that any of the health effects some veterans are experiencing are caused by such exposure' (McAllister, 1998).

Yet, since the goverment had withheld information regarding the release of toxic chemicals from the ammunition dumps, the public distrusted the government's (and even the Presidential Advisory Committee's) findings that there was no proof that there is an organic basis to the Gulf War Syndrome. One eminent spokesperson, for example, called the government's investigations 'irreparably flawed and plagued by arrogant incuriosity and a pervasive myopia that sees a lack of evidence as proof' (Shenon 1997). Accordingly a new panel, independent of the Department of Defense, was recommended (Brown, 1997a).

The syndrome consists of multiple symptoms, the most common of which are chronic fatigue, rash, headache, arthralgias and myalgias, difficulty concentrating, forgetfulness and irritability (Persian Gulf Veterans Coordinating Board, 1995). Subtypes of this illness have been postulated (Brown, 1997b; Haley and Kurt, 1997; Haley *et al.*, 1997a,b; Iowa Persian Gulf Study Group, 1997).

Since the aetiology is uncertain, many have perceived psychogenic causes as likely to be contributory (Amato *et al.*, 1997). Yerkes and Holloway point out, for example, that 'individuals exposed to the uncertainty associated with the Three Mile Island accident had anxiety correlated with elevations of norepinephrine and epinephrine for 10 years and that, similarly, this same sort of phenomenon could have contributed to the Gulf War Syndrome' (Yerkes and Holloway, 1996). Rundell and Ursano cite studies showing that combat veterans with post-traumatic stress disorder (PTSD) have had more somatic symptoms than patients without PTSD in other wars. They conclude that, since stress can impair immunological functioning, the Gulf War Syndrome 'may represent true organic illness or be related to somatic symptom reports after [these] other wars' (Rundell and Ursano, 1996). Further, even if this syndrome is 'delayed' in onset, as Rundell and Ursano postulate above, a psychogenic aetiology may be comparable to the delayed onset of post-traumatic symptoms which has occurred in other wars (Perlman, 1975). Yet servicepersons have not generally been favourably disposed to being told that their symptoms could be wholly or partially psychogenic in origin and caused by stress. Many view this claim as another way in which authorities disrespect them and seek to disown responsibility for the tragic consequences these servicepersons are experiencing. One author, having interviewed several military personnel and discussed with them this possible psychological aetiology, reports, for instance: '*All* of the military personnel that we interviewed were particularly disdainful of this explanation' (emphasis added) (Nicholson *et al.*, 1996).

What, then, should military or civilian careproviders say to these patients, knowing that there is no definitive evidence that their symptoms are organically caused? (Axelrod and Milner, 1997). They could tell them this bluntly. Yet if they do so, some patients may view these careproviders as being in complicity with authorities who fail to appreciate their pain and distress and even, perhaps, wish to deceive them. They may feel outraged at what they take to be the implicit suggestion that their symptoms are, at least in part, psychologically caused. Further, if careproviders share this truth, this alone may destroy the patient–physician relationship.

Alternatively, physicians may say, with comparable truthfulness, that although physical factors have not been determined to be causative with certainty at this time, this remains possible or even likely. This approach is, superficially, clearly preferable. Yerkes and Holloway assert for instance that attributing the symptoms to stress or psychiatric illness is stigmatizing, and that, therefore, the reluctance among careproviders to attribute causality to these factors is appropriate (Yerkes and Holloway, 1996).

Yet there are also potential, albeit highly speculative, risks if careproviders go too far in implying that the likely causes are entirely organic. First, this could result in patients unconsciously using these explanations so that these symptoms become more permanent.

Second, the above risk may be increased if these patients appreciate the decisions made in the Gulf and described above. Namely, they may believe that their symptoms have resulted from the use of 'untested' protective agents and/or the toxic chemicals released from the blown-up ammunition dump. Their symptoms may be worsened by the knowledge that they were caused by the decisions of other persons as opposed to natural events, especially if they believe these persons were negligent in their actions.

Third, as mentioned previously, these patients' symptoms may be exacerbated if they believe that their symptoms have an organic basis, especially if they can anticipate possible secondary gain. It is in fact possible that they may acquire secondary gain from their symptoms if, but only if, they are biologically based. The Presidential Advisory Committee has recommended that 'all 700,000 men and women in the Gulf war veteran population be monitored such that *if there is a plausible biological connection* the secretary would make a presumption of service connection' (emphasis added) (Presidential Advisory Committee, 1996).

Military and civilian doctors, as a result of this situation, face an additional dilemma. Whenever they encounter a person who was in the Gulf and has any symptom which could be part of this syndrome, they must decide whether or not to inform these patients that they should take steps to ensure that the possible connection to their being in the Gulf is recorded.

Fourth—the greatest risk, perhaps—is that many patients might benefit from seeking psychological help, but they may not obtain this help if they believe that their symptoms are wholly organically caused. Psychological interventions in fact may help even if symptoms are entirely physical in origin because they can help patients cope with their impairment.

ANALOGIES WITH OTHER 'POSSIBLY PSYCHOSOMATIC' DISORDERS

When military or civilian doctors treat patients with the Gulf War Syndrome, they are faced with the following dilemma: if they tell these patients that their symptoms may be entirely or partially psychologically based, their patients may become angry and distrust them. 'The mere listing ... [of the Gulf War Syndrome as a possibly psychogenic disorder] ... is likely to infuriate those who have experienced [it] or believe they have' (Micale, 1997). If, on the other hand, they do not tell them this, they are implicitly deceitful.

What, then, should doctors treating these patients do? Should military physicians who know that botulism vaccine was given to some servicepersons without their consent and that some servicepersons may have been exposed to toxic chemicals from the ammunitions dump tell these patients that some consider these possible causative factors, as well?

Fortunately, civilian doctors have been struggling with analogous issues in regard to other illnesses for some time. I believe that one approach more than any other is successful. I describe below first what doctors generally do when treating psychosomatic disorders—the most analogous general group of disorders. I then describe how neurologists treat psychogenic seizures. In discussing this last entity, I describe the approach which has worked the best, and, finally, show how this same approach could be applied to patients with the Gulf War Syndrome.

As stated, an analogous dilemma arises for civilian doctors when they treat patients with psychosomatic disorders. Physicians risk alienating these patients by telling them that their symptoms may be caused by stress or be psychological in origin. Thus, some deceive these patients implicitly by not telling them that the possible aetiology of their symptoms is psychological. Instead, they offer them 'time-limited ... visits independent of physical symptoms', so that by providing this ongoing psychological support, without disclosing what they are doing, they can reduce the patients' symptoms (Margo and Margo, 1994).

This dilemma is also faced by neurologists when they diagnose (and treat) patients with psychogenic seizures. Often, they attempt to make this diagnosis by using a 'sham' procedure, such as seeing if they can elicit a seizure by using a placebo. They may do this without informing the patient, because the patient might find this procedure, like the diagnosis, unacceptable.

Similarly, patients may remain incompletely debriefed because their physicians fear that, if they inform them that their symptoms may be psychologically based, they may respond with anger and shame (Smith *et al.*, 1997). Also, when patients have psychogenic seizures, if their careproviders tell them that their seizures are psychogenic, this typically results in discomfort on the part of the physician. Patients may even terminate the relationship between patient and physician 'as a result of anger and disbelief on the part of the patients' (Benbadis, 1997).

Some neurologists treating patients with psychogenic seizures have, however, had remarkable success in telling them the truth about the possible causes of their disorder. They take great pains to inform these patients initially that, if their symptoms are psychogenically caused, they should not feel that they are of less worth or shame because their careproviders believe that in any case the patients lack 'conscious control over their attacks' (Walczak *et al.*, 1994).

Yet patients may not respond well even if this approach is carried out as conscientiously as possible. Despite the best efforts of clinicians, 'patients' initial understanding and appreciation ... can be overshadowed by ... confusion, embarrassment, and/or defensiveness' (Bortz, 1997). Regardless, this approach may be singularly effective. In one clinic, 'all patients received "comprehensive debriefing" and *none* refused psychotherapy after debriefing' (emphasis added) (Walczak *et al.*, 1994).

What should physicians do, then, when they treat patients with the Gulf War Syndrome? Just as policy makers probably should tell the public the full truth, and even the truth regarding uncertainty after a disaster has occurred, careproviders are also likely to help their patients most by telling them the truth. Since patients' symptoms are unlike disasters, however, in that they may be caused by internal as well as external factors, careproviders must go further when they are responding to individual patients, in addition to telling the truth. Since patients may place different meanings and significance on the possibility that psychological factors have caused or contributed to their symptoms, careproviders must take the initiative to inform patients of the meaning that the careproviders themselves place on this possibility prior to their discussing it. Specifically, careproviders must inform patients that they believe that patients have no more control over developing these symptoms than they would if they were externally caused and, therefore, that these patients are not in any sense at fault.

They should indicate further that though these symptoms may be psychologically caused, they may be as severe or even worse than those caused by physical factors. After the sarin gas attack, as discussed, the St. Luke's Hospital referred to the mental shock these patients might experience as 'terrible' (Komai, 1998). Although it may seem counterintuitive, informing patients accurately regarding the 'worst case scenario' they face may be maximally reassuring. It conveys more genuine empathy. Also, by not understating the extent of the patient's pain, it does not elicit within the patient more elaborate symptoms to prove the careprovider wrong. This latter effect can occur on an unconscious as well as a conscious basis.

A similar approach to patients experiencing the Gulf War Syndrome may, then, also be clinically and ethically the best that can be offered. Military careproviders, having made clear to these patients why they should experience no shame, can then disclose as much about the military's possible contribution to these patients' symptoms as these patients want to know. In so doing, they will not only maximize these patients' outcomes, they will minimize the degree to which they experience ethical conflict in acting as their patients' and the military's agent. Further, they will minimize the degree to which patients might perceive them as serving the military's interests as opposed to their own.

CONCLUSION

Military physicians face ethical problems resulting from conflicting loyalties as do their civilian colleagues. But, due to the military context and its weaponry, the stakes are exponentially higher. In some instances, as a result of these different stakes, the priorities should change, such that military physicians give priority to the needs of the military over those of their patients. The best example of this is military medical triage.

Three examples of this conflict between the duties of military physicians to patients and the military are presented and discussed. Two that arose during the Gulf War are whether military physicians should give servicepersons protective agents without their consent, and when servicepersons should be told that they may have been exposed to toxic chemicals.

The first of these questions involves military physicians' so-called role-specific ethic. According to this concept, military physicians' primary ethical obligation may sometimes be to perform in specific roles whose duties are determined by others and not to make independent decisions themselves. Nonetheless, some suggest that medical authorities in the Gulf who decided to exercise independent judgements chose wisely and by making these judgements in spite of risking greater criticism to themselves, also showed courage.

The second of these questions involves a classic decision between either respecting servicepersons by telling the truth or causing them harm. In this and similar instances, military physicians' practice probably should not deviate substantially from that of their civilian colleagues. They probably should tell the truth, and the whole truth, as soon as this can be done. This decision may not be as costly as some might believe. In addition to respecting servicepersons' dignity, giving immediate accurate information may actually also reduce servicepersons' fear and confusion.

The third ethical dilemma discussed is how physicians, whether military or civilian, should treat servicepersons presenting with the Gulf War Syndrome. The conflict these doctors face between telling these patients the truth and alienating them on one hand, and lying on the other, is discussed. In this instance, as when a catastrophe has occurred, it is preferable to tell the truth, but in this case, since individual patients are involved, that truth alone will not suffice. Before doctors tell these patients the truth that there is no proof now that the cause of their illness is organic, they should inform them how they would view them if their illness were psychologically caused; namely, as not at fault, as feeling comparably at least as severe discomfort and pain, and as having no grounds whatsoever for experiencing shame. By taking this approach, military physicians may be able, in this instance, to serve both their patients' and the military's interests at the same time.

REFERENCES

Amato AA, McVey A, Cha C *et al.* (1997) Evaluation of neuromuscular symptoms in veterans of the Persian Gulf. *Neurology* **48**:4–12.
Axelrod BN and Milner IB (1997) Neurological findings in a sample of Operation Desert Storm veterans. *Journal of Neuropsychiatry and Clinical Neurosciences* **9**:23–28.
Beecher HK (1970) *Research and the Individual/Human Studies*, pp. 209–210. Boston: Little, Brown.
Benbadis SR (1997) Psychogenic seizures. *Neurology* **48**:788.
Binder LM and Rohling ML (1996) Money matters: a meta-analytic review of the effects of financial incentives on recovery after closed-head injury. *American Journal of Psychiatry* **153**:7–10.
Bortz JJ (1997) Nonepileptic seizures: issues in differential diagnosis and treatment. *CNS Spectrums* **2**:20–30.
Brown D (1997a) Independent panel recommended to oversee probe of Gulf War illness. *Washington Post* November 9: A4.
Brown D (1997b) New studies indicate 6 patterns of Gulf 'Syndrome.' *Washington Post* January 9: A1, A11.

Carter BS (1994) Ethical concerns for physicians deployed to operation desert storm. *Military Medicine* **159**:55–59.

Coker WJ (1996) Research/a review of Gulf War illness. *Journal of the Royal Navy Medical Service* **82**:141–146.

Doe v. Sullivan (1991) 938 F. 2d 1370.

Eddington PG and Zaid MS (1997) The true cost of Gulf War Syndrome. *Washington Post* January 1: A19.

Haberman MA (1987) Spontaneous trance as a possible cause for persistent symptoms in the medically ill. *American Journal of Clinical Hypnosis* **29**:171–176.

Haley RW and Kurt TL (1997) Self-reported exposure to neurotoxic chemical combinations in the Gulf War: a cross-sectional epidemiologic study. *Journal of the American Medical Association* **277**:231–237.

Haley RW, Kurt TL and Horn J (1997a) Is there a Gulf War Syndrome? Searching for syndromes by factor analysis of symptoms. *Journal of the American Medical Association* **277**:215–222.

Haley RW, Horn J, Roland PS *et al.* (1997b) Evaluation of neurological function in Gulf War veterans: a blinded case-control study. *Journal of the American Medical Association* **277**:223–230.

Hopkins JET, Stelling HG and Voorhees TS (1969) The marauders and the microbes. In: *Crisis Fleeting* (ed. JH Stone), pp. 293–396. Washington, D.C.: Office of the Surgeon General, Department of the Army.

Howe EG (1986) Ethical issues regarding mixed agency of military physicians. *Social Science and Medicine* **23**:803–815.

Howe EG (1997) Ethical issues in military medicine: mixed agency. In: *Principles and Practice of Military Forensic Psychiatry* (eds RG Lande, DT Armitage), pp. 469–517. Springfield, Ill.: Charles C Thomas.

Howe EG and Martin E (1991) The use of investigational drugs without obtaining servicepersons' consent in the Persian Gulf. *Hastings Center Report* **21**:21–24.

Iowa Persian Gulf Study Group (1997) Self-reported illness and health status among Gulf War veterans: a population-based study. *Journal of the American Medical Association* **277**:238–245.

Jones FD and Koshes RJ (1995) Homosexuality and the military. *American Journal of Psychiatry* **152**:16–21.

Kallen LH, Grodin DM and Vinet RG (1989) Legal aspects of alcohol abuse in the Navy. *Behavioural Sciences and the Law* **7**:355–377.

Komai H (trans) (1995) Sarim gas attack on March 21, 1995. *Asahi Shimbun* newspaper (Available from the author.)

Komai H (1998) Tokyo Subway Sarin Attack, Presentation, September 4. National Naval Medical Center, Bethesda, Maryland.

Margo KL and Margo GM (1994) The problem of somatization in family practice. *American Family Physician* **49**:1873–1879.

McAllister B (1996) Wider gas exposure in Gulf feared. *Washington Post* October 23: A21.

McAllister B (1998) Panel's Report Challenges Gulf War Syndrome Theory. *Washington Post* September 1: A8.

Micale MS (1997) Strange signs of the times. *Times Literary Supplement* May 16: 6–7.

Nicholson GL, Bruton DM and Nicholson NL (1996) Chronic fatigue illness and Operation Desert Storm. *Journal of Occupational and Environmental Medicine* **38**:14–16.

Parrish MD (1962) A veteran of three wars looks at psychiatry in the military. *Psychiatry Opinion* **9**:6–11.

Perlman MS (1975) Basic problems of military psychiatry: delayed reaction in Vietnam veterans. *International Journal of Offender Therapy and Comparative Crimnal Law* **19**:129–138.

Persian Gulf Veterans Coordinating Board (1995) Unexplained illnesses among Desert Storm veterans. *Archives of Internal Medicine* **155**:262–268.

Presidential Advisory Committee on Gulf War Illnesses (1996 Dec) *Final Report*. Washington, DC: US Government Printing Office.

Roberts J (1996) US responds to new suggestion of Gulf War Syndrome. *British Medical Journal* **312**:1629.

Rundell JR and Ursano RJ (1996) Psychiatric responses to war trauma. In: *Emotional Aftermath of the Persian Gulf War* (eds RJ Ursano and AE Norwood), pp. 43–82. Washington, DC: American Psychiatric Association.

Shenon P (1997) House committee assails Pentagon on Gulf War ills. *New York Times* October 26: 1, 18.

Smith ML, Stagno SJ, Dolske M *et al.* (1997) Induction procedures for psychogenic seizures. *Journal of Clinical Ethics* **8**:217–229.

Veatch R (1977) *Case Studies in Medical Ethics*. Cambridge, Ma.: Harvard University Press.

Walczak TS, Williams DT and Berten W (1994) Utility and reliability of placebo infusion in the evaluation of patients with seizures. *Neurology* **44**:394–399.

Yerkes SA and Holloway HC (1996) War and homecomings: the stressors of war and returning from war. In: *Emotional Aftermath of the Persian Gulf War* (eds RJ Ursano and AE Norwood), pp. 25–43. Washington, DC: American Psychiatric Association.

Last things

14

Must We Always Use Advance Directives?

Linda L Emanuel

ABSTRACT

This chapter describes advance directives as one tangible manifestation of the advance care planning process. The process of discourse and planning has a simple goal—to express a patient's prior wishes for use in the event that he or she faces life support decisions and is too ill to participate in decisions. This turns out to be harder to attain than first thought, but other less tangible though important goals have been discovered. The process of seeking an expression of prior wishes, when well done, turns out to have the benefit of bringing the patient and family together with the physician and medical team in a process of adjusting to and coming to terms with the eventuality of dying. The process can make clear to the patient what care and comfort can be offered, can prepare the proxy for his or her role, can bring order to distraught thinking, and generally lend the trust and efficiency to care relationships that comes with a common understanding between members of the team. This essay describes something of how to engage the process, and how not to. It illustrates the approach with three short clinical case analyses.

INTRODUCTION

Three cases introduce this essay.

Case 1
A patient with AIDS and early leucoencephalopathy arrives in the office with his wife and asks to discuss his plans for care when his decision-making capacity fails him. You proceed with the conversation and record his preferences for a couple of likely scenarios; he wants no life-sustaining intervention. Some months later the patient has had personality changes and his insight and rational information use are diminished such that medical decision-making capacity is questionable at best, but he is quite determined in his views. He develops pneumonia with sepsis, and is brought to the emergency room. Now he asks for full intravenous antibiotic treatment and mechanical respiration if necessary.

Case 2

A patient with epilepsy has a living will that asks for no heroic treatment in case of poor prognosis. He suffers a seizure while biking on the bicycle path at the edge of the road and sustains severe head injuries from a resulting collision with a motor vehicle. He enters a comatose state and shows little promise for recovery. His family resist withdrawal of life support despite his advance plans to be allowed to die in such circumstances.

Case 3

A patient with amyotrophic lateral sclerosis has advance care plans that call for avoidance of all life support. Her documents are in the medical record, which has been flagged for their presence. She remains in relatively stable health albeit with decubitus ulcers, still able to work on her fiction writing with computer assistance. She develops a urinary tract infection and then urosepsis. Your colleague, her primary care physician, pursues comfort measures, avoids use of intravenous antibiotics, and calls the family in to inform them that there is a growing likelihood of death. A worried relative calls you to confirm the family's understanding that the advance care plans were not for implementation until the patient became cognitively impaired.

These cases raise many questions, the broadest of which are:

(1) What is advance care planning?
(2) How should it be done, when, and for whom?
(3) What are the risks involved?

This essay first seeks to address these questions in turn, and then turns to the analyses of the above three cases.

WHAT IS ADVANCE CARE PLANNING?

THE GOAL OF ADVANCE CARE PLANNING

Advance care planning is a process of planning medical care in the event that illness involves the patient losing decision-making capacity. Ideally the process is one of continuing discussion, woven integrally into the sequence of clinical encounters (Emanuel *et al.*, 1995). The goals of the process are several. It should help to provide the patient with personal comfort, clarity of thought, and control over the last chapter of his or her life. It should prepare the proxy decision-maker, whether it is the next of kin or someone else, for that role. It should help to guide the physician in decisions that honour the patient's wishes when critically ill. It should also, almost as a side benefit, add understanding, trust and efficiency to decision-making in general between the patient, physician and, when relevant, the family member/proxy. Not insignificantly, it can also help to build the basis for a team of care, in preparation for when the burdens of care are at their highest (Teno *et al.*, 1998).

PROXY DESIGNATION AND INSTRUCTIONAL DIRECTIVES

Advance care planning may result in a written document. This is a useful part of planning because it provides evidence of the patient's wishes. But documentation should not be considered the goal of planning, but rather only as the evidence of wishes. The documentation should aim to be a true reflection of the patient's intent, expressed in such a way that it is a useful guide in making clinical decisions.

Planning falls conceptually into two broad categories. A person may choose a proxy decision-maker, also termed 'a durable power of attorney for health care' in the United States. The purpose of a proxy is to serve in the role of patient, discussing medical decisions with the physician as the patient would have. Often, patients will choose a loved one as the proxy. Due to the burden of being a proxy, and due to the potential for emotional or fiscal differences of interest between the patient and the loved one, it is sometimes better to choose a more distant friend or official person (Emanuel and Emanuel, 1992). A proxy's role may be interpreted in three different ways. It may be to carry out the patient's explicit prior wishes about treatment as precisely as possible. It may be to attempt a balance between the patient's interests and the needs of others, interpreting all these in the context that arises much as the patient would have or even with unmodified use of the proxy's own judgement (Lynn, 1991). Or it may be to make an assessment of the patient's best interests and advocate only for these. It is helpful if a patient can guide the proxy ahead of time regarding which of these interpretations he or she favours.

A patient may also provide directives regarding his or her wishes. Patients using this approach may write down their wishes. The written document can be completed in a variety of ways, ranging from a free-prose letter to a simple 'living will' form or a validated questionnaire form or medical directive. Written documents are most useful if they include a validated questionnaire form, since these have undergone rigorous procedures in design and testing that evidence the scope, meaning, fairness in framing and relevance of the questions (Alpert *et al.*, 1996). Validated forms are most likely, by definition, to cover the relevant issues, provide a true reflection of the patient's views, and provide them in a form that can be used clinically. Such directives tend to include a patient's overall values, goals for care in specified scenarios, and a sample of specific treatment choices for those scenarios (Patrick *et al.*, 1997).

For the great majority of patients it is helpful to use both modalities, designating someone to be a proxy and providing the physician and proxy with guidance as to the patient's wishes. Occasionally a patient will have no one suitable to designate as a proxy; such a person may do well with an instructional approach and no proxy, leaving the physician as the sole patient advocate. Occasionally the reverse will occur—the patient can name a proxy but has too much difficulty imagining future scenarios. Wherever possible, patients should be encouraged to both have a proxy and provide instructions.

WHICH DOCUMENTS?

Documents can be divided into advisory and statutory (Emanuel, 1995). Advisory documents aim to reflect the patient's wishes as accurately as possible, and these are legal under constitutional law as an expression of the patient's wishes. Those that are statutory aim to provide some protection against litigation for the physician who follows a patient's wishes, whether those wishes are to withdraw or withhold life-sustaining intervention or to use it. Advisory documents are most useful if they have been designed to reliably reflect the relevant wishes of the patient; that is, if they have been validated. Statutory documents should comply with statutory law (Right to Die Legislation, 1994). In the United States, compliance may be with state law or with uniform standards. Some documents combine an advisory section with statutory requirements, saving the physician and patient the trouble of using two forms together.

JUSTIFYING PRINCIPLES AND LIMITATIONS OF ADVANCE CARE PLANNING

In some sense advance care planning is little different from estate planning for the possibility of accident or death. In both situations, individuals are extending their autonomy beyond the time when they can execute it for themselves. The notion is one of surviving interest; that is, interests which survive beyond one's ability to secure them directly.

As with all clinical interventions, advance care planning has limits to its applicability. An easy (and optimistic) confusion is to think that advance care planning can solve the common problem of how to honour the wishes of a patient with dementia. Advance care planning, as the argument would have it, provides authentic wishes for that patient. Unfortunately, this is not so. Advance care planning is justified as real-time wishes for a future circumstance when there are no other wishes that can be honoured, as is the case with estate planning. If a person has wishes, albeit demented wishes, it is not so clear that prior wishes trump the real-time wishes (Dresser, 1989). So, advance care planning can be one guide among others as to what would be in the best interest of a dementia patient, but it does not have conclusive authority. Full authority of prior wishes occurs only in cases where the patient is comatose or so ill that there can be no reasonable expectation that he or she has any wishes at all. In neurology, where central nervous system involvement is quite common, this is an important point.

HOW SHOULD IT BEST BE DONE?

INITIATING THE PROCESS

The process of advance care planning can be initiated as a routine matter while the patient is in good health. Brochures and worksheets in waiting areas, informational videos and patient resource groups are all helpful. Physicians may raise the topic as a regular matter along with other aspects of routine check-ups. Physician involvement in these cases largely falls to primary care physicians.

The neurologist may not see a patient until central nervous system damage has already made it meaningless to initiate advance care planning. When a neurologist receives a patient referral from a primary care physician it is important to know whether advance care planning has occurred. If so, the neurologist should receive both the documentation and the contact information of the physician who was involved in the planning so that in the event of patient incompetence there is a maximal chance that his or her wishes are applied well to the circumstances at hand.

If no advance care planning has occurred for a decision-incapacitated patient, the neurologist may still find it helpful to go through the process of advance care planning with the family for the purposes of building a care team relationship that is prepared for good decision-making. Naturally the documentation will not have the binding nature of a patient's prior wishes, but the clarity may be useful nonetheless.

A CORE STRUCTURED DISCUSSION

The core discussion is most important, and is most efficiently done by going through a worksheet or validated questionnaire form that can later be used as an advisory document (Emanuel, 1993). This can have been given to the patient ahead of time, and the physician should suggest that the patient arrive at the next visit having gone through the worksheet. It is also very helpful to have the patient bring a potential proxy. Then, going through the worksheet briefly together, the physician can explain relevant medical features of the scenarios and treatment options, and review the patient's choices. The physician should check to see that the patient is making choices that are consistent with the patient's own goals, medically sensible, and within the physician's and proxy's range of moral acceptability.

REVIEW

Advance care planning documents are inhibiting to many patients if they are seen as static and permanently binding. Patients may change their minds and are free to change their documents at any time as long as they retain decision-making competence. Conversations about future illness are often comfortable once the first core discussion has occurred. This longitudinal discourse may reveal changes in a patient's disposition. In addition, it is helpful to review advance care planning periodically. This may occur when a major life event occurs or as soon as the changes are settled, whether that event is a change in health status, a marriage, a divorce, a birth, a bereavement or an experience that alters the patient's views about medical care. In the absence of such change routine review is a good idea, say every five years.

APPLICATION

When a patient has become decision-incapacitated, and life-sustaining intervention is medically appropriate, the task is to fit the prior wishes to the circumstances (Emanuel *et al.*, 1994). Application of wishes can be difficult if the wishes were not well stated (Schneiderman *et al.*, 1992; Fischer *et al.*, 1997). For instance, an expression that simply states a desire for no heroic treatment in case of poor prognosis does not help the physician or proxy understand what the patient would consider heroic treatment or poor prognosis; in such cases advance directives may be of no help (Eisendrath and Jonsen, 1983). Poorly stated advance directives may also be seriously misinterpreted. For instance, a patient who wishes to avoid permanent ventilator dependence may risk denial of temporary respiratory assistance for a reversible condition if the advance directive contains only a generic statement to avoid ventilator use.

WHAT ARE THE RISKS?

UNJUSTIFIED ASSUMPTIONS

The presence of documented advance care planning should not be assumed to mean that a patient wants to forgo life-sustaining intervention. Advance care planning is supposed to be a portrait of the patient's wishes, whether they are for aggressive intervention, comfort care or something intermediate.

Another misunderstanding involves the circumstances under which an advance care planning document comes into play. In the great majority of cases, the authority of the proxy starts when the patient loses decision-making capacity, and not before (Appelbaum *et al.*, 1987). The authority of written wishes in an advance directive is also absent so long as the patient has real-time decision-making capacity. In addition, full authenticity of written prior wishes occurs only when the patient is incapable of real-time wishes.

CASE ANALYSES

Case 1

As described above, in this case a patient has had personality changes and lacks decision-making capacity but has definite wishes which differ from his documented prior wishes.

The justifying principle for advance care planning is that of a person's surviving interests. This case falls only partially into that sphere of justification. The patient's personality changes make it unclear whether the wishes of the pre-illness personality or the real-time personality take precedence (Dresser, 1989). Four considerations may assist the physician and proxy as they decide how much weight to give the prior wishes, present wishes, the proxy's substituted judgement, and the patient's best interest.

First, if it were clear that the illness directly caused altered and unsound judgement (for instance by having caused a confusional state) it might be that the proxy and physician must 'side with' the healthy personality, in this case the prior personality.

Second, if the new disposition appears to reflect a change of heart that is not directly illness generated it is more defensible to see the present person as authentic and honour the most recent wishes, as with a circumstance and decision for a decision-capacitated patient.

The third possibility is to estimate the best substituted judgement by asking how operative the patient's wish would be if decision-making capacity were intact. When individuals make rational decisions, many wishes may be acknowledged and then balanced with features of the circumstance. So some wishes of a patient without decision-making capacity may weigh more heavily than they would for that same real-time personality if the full balancing of intact decision-making were to occur. In this case, would the desire to live still outweigh other desires and competing considerations if the patient could compute them all?

The fourth possibility is to estimate what would be in the best interests of the patient. This estimate may seem obviously to live as long as possible. But many consider their legacy their greatest interest. So the proxy must also consider how the use of life-sustaining intervention might impact on the memory of the patient and his legacy in general.

In this case the analysis varies depending on the above considerations; the physician and proxy must work together to consider which aspects of the patient's wishes and current personality are to be honoured. There is one clearly generalizable feature about this case: prior wishes do not necessarily trump the patient's real-time wishes.

Case 2

In this case a family wants a course of action that the patient did not want.

In the absence of a specific proxy designation, the next of kin may take that role and may have de facto authority in medical decision-making, equivalent to that which the patient would have had. However, in this case there is a written instruction from the patient, and it has the full authority of the patient's prior wishes since the patient is now comatose and unable either to have a wish or to make a decision. If the patient had no prior discussion with his family it is hard to know how much, if any, latitude he would have wanted to allow for the family's different wishes. So, unless the family has good reason to believe that the written instruction is not fully authentic, the physician should explain to the family that the living will is taken to be the best evidence of the patient's wishes and those wishes should be honoured.

It is documented in several studies that proxy decision-making may not track the wishes of the patient (Emanuel and Emanuel, 1992). This is especially true when the patient's wishes are to allow death. There are two likely reasons for discrepancy. The burden of living with a decision that allows death is great, and proxies are understandably averse to decision regret. It is hard to let go of a loved one and especially hard when the loss is sudden and there has been little preparatory discussion and time to adjust to mortality. It can be helpful for the physician to acknowledge these difficulties and to give the family some time to adjust. But the acknowledgement and time should allow for overcoming the difficulties rather than bowing to them. In this case, the patient's wishes should be honoured.

The complicating feature here is that the living will may be variously interpreted. It was not a well-validated instructional directive but a general statement that did not guide the family or physician regarding the patient's interpretation of heroic measures or poor prognosis. The family could logically argue that, while life exists and technology is available, life-sustaining measures are not heroic. They could also argue that, where life exists and miracles are possible, the prognosis might improve. Such an interpretation is unlikely in this situation, and the family should not be invited to think this way.

Case 3

This patient is mentally competent but unable to communicate directly. Her advance care planning wishes are treated as though they were already in effect.

It is hard for any second party to communicate with a patient who has ALS sufficiently advanced that speech and facial expressions are lost. (This patient might benefit from having a prominent sign by her at all times stating something like: 'My mind works fine, only my muscles don't—please read my computer response to talk with me'.) It can also be hard for physicians (and others) to talk about plans for care when death is a real possibility. It can also be hard to recognize and deal with a physician's occasional internal sense that maybe it would be better for the patient to die.

In this case, though, the advance care plans have no standing whatsoever, since the patient is fully mentally competent. The physician makes a mistake to follow the advance directives. The patient has a means of communication using her computer, and full efforts must be made to discuss with the patient what she wants (Appelbaum *et al.*, 1987).

SUMMARY

In summary, advance care planning is a process of discussion, intended to clarify and unify expectations and goals for care in case of mental incapacity. It can also help achieve general comfort with mortality and with shared decision-making, for the physician and the patient and indeed for the proxy. A written document may be evidence of the patient's wishes and can be helpful if it is well drafted. In many cases, and especially among neurology patients, there are pitfalls to be aware of. In particular, the three cases of this chapter have illustrated three points. Prior wishes do not trump all current wishes, even for decision-incapacitated patients. Proxy or family decision-making can take different forms, but in general the patient's prior wishes take priority over the family/proxy wishes. Prior wishes have no standing if the patient is still mentally competent. Despite the possible pitfalls, advance care planning is a useful skill in the practice of medicine, aiding respect for patients' wishes, and its proper use should be encouraged.

REFERENCES

Alpert H, Hoijtink H, Fischer G and Emanuel LL (1996) Psychometric analysis of an advance directive. *Medical Care* **34**:1057–1065.

Appelbaum PS, Lidz CW and Meisel A (1987) *Informed Consent: Legal Theory and Clinical Practice.* New York: Oxford University Press.

Dresser RS (1989) *Advance Directives in Medicine*, pp. 155–170. New York: Praeger.

Eisendrath SJ and Jonsen AR (1983) The living will: help or hindrance? *New England Journal of Medicine* **249**:2054.

Emanuel LL (1993) Advance directives: what have we learned so far? *Journal of Clinical Ethics* **4(1)**:8–16.

Emanuel LL (1995) Advance directives. In: *Principles and Practice of Supportive Oncology* (eds A Gerger *et al.*). Philadelphia: Lippincott-Raven.

Emanuel EJ and Emanuel LL (1992) Proxy decision making. *Journal of the American Medical Association* **267**:2221–2226.

Emanuel LL, Barry MJ, Stoeckle JD and Emanuel EJ (1994) Advance directives: extrapolation to unstated decisions. *Medical Care* **32**:95–105.

Emanuel LL, Danis M, Pearlman RA and Singer PA (1995) Advance care planning as a process. *Journal of the American Geriatric Society* **43**:440–446.

Fischer GS, Alpert HR, Stoeckle JD and Emanuel LL (1997) Can goals of care be used to predict intervention preferences in an advance directive? *Archives of Internal Medicine* **157**:801–807.

Lynn J (1991) Why I don't have a living will. *Law and Medical Health Care* **9**:101–104.

Patrick DL, Pearlman RA, Starks HE *et al.* (1997) Validation of preference for life-sustaining treatment: implications for advance care planning. *Annals of Internal Medicine* **127**:509–517.

Right to Die Legislation (1994). New York: Choice in Dying.

Schneiderman LJ, Pearlman RA, Kaplan RM *et al.* (1992) Relationship of general advance directive instructions to specific life-sustaining treatment preferences in patients with serious illness. *Archives of Internal Medicine* **152**:2114–2122.

Teno JM, Stevens M, Spernak S and Lynn J (1998) Role of written advance directives in decision-making. *Journal of General Internal Medicine* **13**:439–446.

15

When, If Ever, Should Treatment be Withdrawn?

Christopher D Ward

ABSTRACT

Eight ethical maxims are helpful in deciding whether treatment should be discontinued:

(1) A medical decision should primarily serve the patient's best interests.
(2) The patient's known preferences must be respected unless there are strong ethical reasons for disregarding them.
(3) Expressed preferences are not an infallible guide to the patient's long-term wishes.
(4) The interests of others must sometimes prevail over the patient's preferences.
(5) Conflicting interests are judged by assessing the patient's rights in relation to the rights of others.
(6) Compassion should influence decisions but must not negate justice.
(7) The patient is a person with whom doctors and professionals have a special relationship.
(8) No brain damage is severe enough to remove the doctor's obligation to regard the patient as a person and to serve that individual's best interests.

A decision based on these maxims will be consistent with English law and professional codes. It will be biased towards the patient and towards the patient's best interests, although other factors will be relevant. It is important to determine who is *qualified* to be involved in the decision (sometimes as a surrogate for the patient) and who is *competent* to be involved.

INTRODUCTION

Neurologists are often involved with a decision to reduce or discontinue treatment either because it is considered to be ineffective (and perhaps costly), or because the treatment is thought to be prolonging life without bringing any benefits to the patient. This essay examines some of the principles which can be used to guide the decision and concludes with some comments on a related question: who can make the decision?

GIVING DEATH A CHANCE

Most would agree that there are situations in which treatment should be discontinued. The purpose of medical treatment is to serve the best interests of the patient, and very few patients would always regard staying alive as in their best interests. From a Christian perspective, Dietrich Bonhoeffer's remarks on bodily life are probably typical: life must be protected against arbitrary killing, but need not be preserved in *all* circumstances (Bonhoeffer, 1963). By excepting 'extraordinary means of treatment' from the duty to preserve life, Pope Pius XII in 1957 clearly indicated that medical care was not to be motivated by an over-riding concern for life at any cost. Anglo-American law takes a similar position. The House of Lords' ruling on the discontinuance of nutritional support for someone with severe brain damage stated that 'this principle [the sanctity of life], fundamental though it is, is not absolute' (Airdale NHS Trust v. Bland, 1993).*

There are circumstances in which most doctors would be likely to 'pull out all the stops', for example if a young patient becomes acutely ill. In others they are more likely to 'give death a chance', to use Weir's phrase (1989, p. 335). The basis for these distinctions should be scrutinized. Is one life perceived as more valuable than another? What is the logical basis for offering different levels of 'routine medical care' to different patients (for example different doses or routes of administration of antibiotics), as though death were being offered a better chance in some circumstances than in others? The intuition that a doctor is less responsible for acts of omission than for acts of commission is logically questionable (Harris, 1985). Decisions about reducing or withdrawing treatment are rarely easy but the next two sections aim to show how they can be made more transparent.

WINNERS AND LOSERS IN MEDICAL DECISION-MAKING

Table 15.1 shows that, in addition to the patient, health care decisions affect many other parties, including the family or friends of the patient, professionals, the health care system and society at large. The matrix is further complicated when the patient is unable to participate in decision-making.

The factors listed in Table 15.1 are often in conflict with one another. For example, withdrawing treatment may benefit the patient but cause the family overwhelming guilt. Professionals also have concerns which are distinct from

---

* For a discussion of this and other cases, see McHale *et al.* (1977).

Table 15.1   Benefits and risks of withdrawing treatment when benefits are minimal

	Benefits of discontinuing treatment	Harmful effects of discontinuing treatment
For the person (whether or not able to express wishes)	Benefits of treatment outweighed by present or anticipated suffering	Deprived of opportunity for unanticipated recovery If recovery unexpectedly occurs, patient may not be offered rehabilitation because of poor prognosis
For the non-autonomous person	Incapacity to express wishes may render life not worth living to many people	Wishes may have been misrepresented If recovery unexpectedly occurs, potential damage to relationships with family and doctors
For the family	Fulfilling the duty to respect person's wishes Compassionate response to suffering	Neglect of duty to loved person; violation of love; ensuing guilt
For society	Economy of resources where benefits are marginal; justice	Setting dangerous precedents which could threaten society
For professionals	Fulfilling the duty to respect person's wishes Economy of professional resources Fulfilling duty to society as a whole	Potential neglect of duty of care Potential for harming patient Potential legal repercussions

those of the patient, for example the risk of exposure to litigation if treatment is withheld (although a doctor should not delay or alter treatment merely because of personal risk [GMC, 1995]). Competing claims on health care resources produce tensions between the individual and society. Other tensions arise from society's interest in upholding its collective moral values and in preventing its more powerful members—including doctors—from harming vulnerable people, for example by taking life-and-death decisions without consulting them.

Many different criteria are deployed to resolve conflicts. We use moral criteria to assess the balance of harm and benefit and to evaluate the interests of patients and of family members. In addition professionals are constrained by codes of professional conduct. Other non-moral criteria, for example guidelines laid down by a local health authority, may also influence decisions to discontinue expensive treatments (see Chapter 9). There is also a further set of statutory and common-law constraints on professionals and patients. Moreover, many people, including professionals, conceive of their own preferences as balanced not only against those of other people but against externally imposed rules: a professional wishes to relieve the patient of suffering but withdrawal of treatment contravenes a moral code; a family is prevented from agreeing to treatment (for example blood transfusion) for religious reasons.

USING THEORIES TO SUPPORT DECISIONS

Western medical ethics can be seen as based on the four classic principles of beneficence (doing good), non-maleficence (avoiding doing harm), autonomy, and justice (Gillon, 1986) (see Essay 10 for further comments on autonomy). Decision-makers need to operationalize these principles; they cannot rely only on intuition to yield optimal solutions. Brody (1988) discusses five ethical appeals: to the consequences of a decision; to rights; to respect for persons; to virtues (for example, compassion); and to cost-effectiveness and justice. I will use these as the basis for eight maxims which can be used to create rules to support health care decision-making.

Maxim 1: *A medical decision should primarily serve the patient's best interests*
The idea that medicine must serve the best interests of the patient, enshrined both in professional codes (GMC, 1995) and in the law (F v. West Berkshire HA, 1989), is based on the appeal to consequences. The ethical appeal to consequences is utilitarian in character: whatever produces the best practical results is the best decision. However, there are consequences for the family and for society as well as for the patient (see Maxim 4), which is why the patient's best interests cannot be paramount in all circumstances.

> **Case example 1**
> Mrs M, a woman of 48, develops pneumonia following successive middle cerebral artery infarcts in both hemispheres, a few weeks apart. She has a past history of severe depression with repeated suicide attempts, and alcoholism. The neurologist is considering discontinuing treatment but her husband insists that 'everything possible should be done' to treat her pneumonia. The physician who previously treated the medical complications of her alcoholism also advocates aggressive treatment on the grounds that there is a slim chance of a satisfactory outcome.

There is evidence that Mrs M might have found life scarcely worth living prior to the series of strokes, and it is clear that she can expect severe cognitive and physical disability if she survives. Assessing her best interests would entail balancing the possible benefits of extending her life against the negative consequences of remaining alive. It is arguable that her best interests might not be served by continuing the treatment for pneumonia, notwithstanding her husband's view. Medical opinion (from the neurologist and the physician) can help to predict the likely outcome for Mrs M. The courts have often relied on doctors to assess the patient's best interests (Bolan v. Friern Barnet HMC, 1957).

However, such matters are not fully within the doctors' field of expertise: a life which does not seem worth living to the doctor may be valued by the patient.

Maxim 2: *The patient's known preferences must be respected unless there are strong ethical reasons for disregarding them*
One criterion for judging outcomes is the extent to which the patient's preferences are satisfied. In the case of a non-autonomous patient an advance directive (living will) may give us evidence of preferences concerning the use of aggressive medical treatment in critical illness. Alternatively the evidence of family or friends might establish the patient's likely preferences.

> Mrs M (see above) is aphasic and cannot express a view about whether treatment should be continued but her sister and other relatives report that she has often dreaded the prospect of becoming 'a vegetable'. They believe that her preference would be for treatment to be discontinued.

Even in the absence of a written advance directive, evidence concerning Mrs M's preferences should be taken into account.

> **Case example 2**
> An obese man of 35 with spina bifida and an IQ in the low-normal range has a large sacral skin sore. There are early signs of osteomyelitis and a high risk of a potentially fatal septicaemia. The sore could be healed by a rigorous programme including intravenous antibiotics, calorie restriction and prolonged bed rest. He is certain that with prolonged hospitalization he would lose his job. He declines the offer of hospital treatment, although it is made clear to him that returning to work will pose a serious health risk.

Physicians and other professionals can often see that a particular course of action is the optimal way of serving a patient's best interests and are tempted to impose their views on patients. It is arguable that hospital treatment is in this man's 'best interests' (Maxim 1), but his own preference must prevail (Maxim 2).

Maxim 3: *Expressed preferences are not an infallible guide to the patient's long-term wishes*
We often doubt whether the patient's expressed preference serves his best interests. Patients' views of what they might benefit from are not always a trustworthy guide to the outcomes they would in fact most value. We need to establish the patient's ability to understand the issues and to express preferences which are consistent with his other longer-term wishes and dispositions (see Appendix for the Law Commission's [1995] criteria for determining the patient's best interests). We should clearly distrust preferences which appear to be impulsive and insubstantial, for example when a severely injured patient's demand for treatment to be discontinued is a manifestation of depression. However, we should be cautious when using Maxim 3 to override Maxim 2.

The team looking after the man with spina bifida was faced with the dilemma that his immature personality and low intelligence might have impeded him from making the best decision. Was his expressed preference compatible with his long-term aspirations? They concluded that he was sufficiently competent to make his own decisions; in adults, there is a high threshold for deeming someone incompetent. I return to the issue of competence later.

Maxim 4: *The interests of others must sometimes prevail over the patient's preferences*

A person's wishes must sometimes be disregarded because they would be unjust to others, for example if a patient requests continuance of a very costly treatment considered by the doctor to be ineffective. In practice the health care team typically has little evidence on which to base a realistic judgement of costs. However, in R. v. Cambridge DHA (1995) the principle was accepted, both in the High Court and more explicitly in the Court of Appeal, that the equitable use of health care resources was relevant to a health authority's decision not to fund treatment for a child with leukaemia. Cost was also taken into consideration in Airdale NHS Trust v. Bland (1993).

Maxim 5: *Conflicting interests are judged by assessing the patient's rights in relation to the rights of others*

A useful way of thinking about the principle of justice is in terms of rights; that is, the obligations owed by others. The decision to discontinue treatment must take account of the patient's right not to be killed, to be aided when ill, to participate in health care decisions, and to receive a medical second opinion (BMA, 1992; GMC, 1995). Some of the philosophical and legal issues related to rights are complex but it is uncontroversial that people have obligations towards one another. Some obligations are enshrined in law, some are endorsed by social custom, and some are construed privately between individuals. The reciprocal of an obligation is a right (Brody, 1988). Cost considerations arise because the NHS has statutory obligations to all its patients, and doctors have moral and professional obligations to others whose rights must be respected. Conflicts between the interests of family members and the patient can be understood in a similar way. The personal interests of individual professionals are also relevant, for example when a patient's wish to end life is morally unacceptable to a physician. The physician has the right to refuse to provide treatment she considers inappropriate (Re J (A minor) (Medical treatment), 1992) although she has a duty to explain to a patient how her beliefs may affect treatment decisions (GMC, 1995).

The function of Maxim 5 is to clarify the process of weighing up the rights and obligations of all those with a stake in treatment decisions. The husband of Mrs M (the woman with multiple strokes, depression and alcoholism) feels that he is discharging a moral obligation to his wife by insisting on her receiving maximum treatment. On the other hand the neurologist has an obligation to Mrs M to act in her best interests. The neurologist may have a conscientious objection to providing further treatment which will result in months or years of misery for Mrs M, and may have the right not to provide treatment. However, Mrs M's husband could appeal to his wife's right to receive medical care. Other patients could suffer if Mrs M's hospital treatment is prolonged and expensive, and their rights should also be entered into the equation.

Provided we are confident of the patient's true wishes, and provided we can weigh up the strength of the obligations owed to her against the strength of obligations owed to others, Maxims 1 to 5 provide a framework for assessing consequences justly. However, many professionals recoil from this essentially utilitarian approach because it fails to capture the essence of the dilemmas they usually face. A compassionate impulse is likely to overthrow the decision in either direction: discontinuing a costly treatment may seem cruel or, in other circumstances, preserving a life could seem equally cruel.

Maxim 6: *Compassion should influence decisions but must not negate justice*
Compassion, the most powerful of the appeals to virtue (Brody, 1988), can tip the balance in favour of a course of action but should not totally subvert the process of rational decision-making.

> **Case example 3**
> Two years after suffering severe cerebral anoxia following a trauma to the right carotid artery, a woman of 32 is still attending physiotherapy twice weekly, as well as receiving monthly speech therapy sessions. She has extremely limited cognitive and communicative abilities, severely impaired sitting and standing balance, no independent mobility, and no objective evidence of improvement for the previous year. Her mother still firmly believes that she is progressing, has given up her career to be able to provide care, and unfailingly attends every therapy session. The decision to continue treatment is motivated by compassion for the patient, and especially for her mother. Meanwhile other patients are having to wait 6 months for outpatient therapy appointments.

Compassionate motivation must be weighed against other valid moral or legal considerations. Compassion is a freely given additional benefit, not a tax enforced on others. Unfair distribution of scarce health care resources is not compassionate: Robin Hood would not have been compassionate if he had robbed the poor to give to the poor. The main function of Maxim 6 is to place *limits* on the compassionate impulse. However, compassion does have a proper role in decision-making through the next maxim, which concerns the privileged status of the patient in relation to the professionals who are treating him.

Maxim 7: *The patient is a person with whom physicians and professionals have a special relationship.*
The appeal to respect for persons is fundamental. As Frankfurt (1971) says, concepts of personhood 'are designed to capture those attributes which are ... the source of what we regard as most important and most problematic in our lives'. Physicians should aim to maximize the dignity, integrity and autonomy of an individual. There would have to be strong reasons for subjecting patients to treatments which were physically or psychologically degrading, *even if the patient chose them.* One role for respect of the person in deciding whether to discontinue treatment is essentially an appeal to rights: a human body—any

member of the human species—has minimal legal rights but the moral obligations owed to a person, the claimable rights, are perhaps greater. The appeal to persons is a sort of aide memoire—this is not merely a body, but has the status of a person.

A crucial property of a person is the capacity for relationships with other persons. The responsibilities which people bear towards one another are proportional to the strengths of their inter-relationships: for example, a woman has stronger obligations to her child than to her employer. The patient–physician relationship, a key concept in the GMC's professional code (1995), places special obligations on the physician. The existence of a personal relationship between a professional and a patient biases the professional towards the interests of that individual rather than towards the interests of other people. The relationship is also the channel through which compassion can be expressed.

Case example 4

A man aged 64 with severe motor neurone disease is keen to continue receiving an expensive drug treatment although there is little evidence that it will alter the long-term outcome. There are other patients whose claim to receive the drug is marginally better. The Health Authority queries the continued use of the treatment but the neurologist defends its use.

The neurologist's arguments include: (a) that there is *some* evidence that drug treatment is in the best interests of the patient (Maxim 1); (b) the patient wants the treatment (Maxim 2). The interests of others (Maxim 5) marginally outweigh those of the patient, but compassion (Maxim 6) and the special status of the patient in the patient–physician relationship (Maxim 7) give the neurologist a good case for continuing treatment.

Maxim 8: *No brain damage is severe enough to remove the doctor's obligation to regard the patient as a person and to serve that person's best interests*
The Law Commission judges best interests primarily in terms of the principle of autonomy and the appeal to respect for persons (Law Commission, 1995; see Appendix). However, these principles can seem hollow when deciding on the further treatment of someone in a persistent vegetative state (PVS). We may consider (with Brody, 1988) that the obligations we owe to individuals *as persons* vary from case to case. Perhaps the potential personhood of an individual in PVS is so diminished as to have little influence on a treatment decision. However, I believe such an approach to personhood to be unworkable. Judging a patient to be less than a full person deprives us of a crucial criterion for making decisions: an individual who has lost personhood can hardly have 'best interests' of the kind invoked in the House of Lords' ruling on Anthony Bland's nutrition and hydration (Airdale NHS Trust v. Bland, 1993).

Dworkin (1977) has suggested that 'rights are trumps': like trump cards, they have more force than any other considerations. This is not true of all the rights/obligations pairings I have discussed here, but it is true of the right to be respected as a person. Judgements about the degree of personhood of those who are confused or cognitively impaired are philosophically and ethically dubious and contravene the right to be treated as a person in all circumstances. In other words, Maxim 8 is inviolable.

The patient's family and friends often have a very different view from that of the professionals. The social person is to some extent *constructed* by those who have loved him and love him still. Relatives who impute purpose to the random eye movements of someone with severe brain damage also impute meaning to the individual as a person with wishes and potentialities. Whatever the factual rights and wrongs of their perceptions (and relatives are not wrong in every instance), I suggest that professionals are morally obliged to respect the person as perceived by others. However, respect for the person also entails having a view on that person's best interests, which may not be served by remaining alive.

> **Case example 5**
> A farmer's wife with MS was receiving treatment for pneumonia. She had very little voluntary movement. She was severely demented, visual impairment was so severe that she could not watch or understand a television programme, and she was doubly incontinent with recurrent skin sores. Her devoted husband was asked whether he thought active treatment was in her best interests. He replied 'Do whatever is needed, doctor, provided she does not end as a cabbage'. The doctor was shocked by this response: he had not appreciated how this woman's severely restricted life was perceived by her loving family.

Figure 15.1 necessarily oversimplifies the considerations which contribute to decisions on continuing or discontinuing treatment but it brings out the main points encapsulated in the maxims. The patient is in a privileged position (a) because professionals owe him more consideration than they owe to other involved parties such as the family, society and themselves, and (b) for the related reason that the patient can benefit from compassion. Professionals are not mandated to be compassionate but they have a moral obligation to relieve suffering. These two factors bias treatment decisions in favour of the patient's best interests but they do not totally override the interests of others.

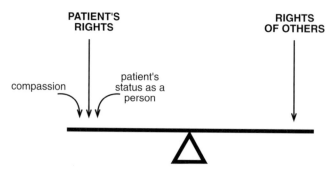

Figure 15.1   The balance between the rights and obligations of the patient and others: the relationship between the patient and professionals biases the decision towards the patient's best interests.

WHO CAN DECIDE IF AND WHEN TO WITHDRAW TREATMENT?

There are two questions to answer here. First, who is qualified to be involved in a decision? Second, who is competent to be involved? The patient is always qualified to be involved but may or may not be competent. As we have seen, others such as family members and professionals also have legitimate interests in the decision to withdraw treatment but they vary in their competence to contribute effectively to decision-making.

The third clause of the Law Commission's standards for acting in a patient's best interests (Law Commission, 1995; see Appendix) requires us to establish which of the four types of decision-maker listed in Table 15.1 are qualified to participate in deciding whether to withdraw treatment (second clause, op. cit.). The patient clearly has the (waivable) right to be involved if at all possible, even if she is not fully competent to make a decision. Equally, the responsible physician must be involved in the decision in all circumstances. This sounds obvious, but I agree with McLean (1994) that medical opinion in decision-making has been overvalued by society and by the courts. The physician is not the final arbiter on the issues summarized in Figure 15.1 although she has important roles in meeting the Law Commission's criteria for acting in the patient's best interests (Law Commission, 1995; Appendix). The physician's tasks are (1) to assess the competence of the patient; (2) to provide information about risks and benefits of treatment to assist the patient and family to reach a decision; (3) to indicate whether a suggested course of action is professionally and morally acceptable to her; and (4) to represent to the patient and family the issues relating to cost and justice. A nurse and sometimes one or more other professionals must often be involved for similar reasons, and also because the reasoning behind the decision must be clearly understood by the whole professional team.

Unless the patient can choose them, it is more difficult to establish which family members or friends should be involved in the decision to withdraw treatment. The degree of closeness to the patient is often difficult to assess: emotional links do not necessarily coincide with kinship. Where the interests of relatives are thought to be in conflict with those of the patient an advocate for the patient such as a social worker should be included. Occasionally, for example in a court hearing, society at large is represented in the discussions about discontinuing treatment. Some method of disentangling clinical decision-making from considerations of cost and justice would be useful in many other situations. As a Massachusetts judge put it: 'such questions of life and death seem to us to require the process of detached but passionate investigation and decision that forms the ideal on which the judicial branch of government was created' (Weir, 1989, p. 112).

The other question to consider is the competence of the decision-makers in reaching a decision which is (a) in the best interests of the patient, and (b) just. All the participants in the decision (including the patient, if he is capable of being involved) face similar questions: have the patient's enduring values and preferences (rather than transient feelings) been properly understood? Have the most likely alternative outcomes been correctly conceived (not just short-term but longer-term outcomes)?

According to Buchanan and Brock (1989), tests of competency divide people into those whose decisions are binding and those whose decisions should be set aside. This holds true for many potential decision-makers, but many patients are in an intermediate position because their competence is compromised, for example by brain damage. Such patients can *participate* in the decision-making process, assisting but not fully determining it. The simple tests of verbal memory and of verbal communication which are conventionally used to screen patients give only partial answers to the question of competency in decision-making and indeed there is no absolute standard. For patients who are conscious but confused, professional skill and ingenuity are needed to confirm their level of comprehension and their preferences. Even if family members and friends are eminently qualified to act as surrogates they may not be competent to do so. Their ability to comprehend the current situation and the possible outcomes, and to place themselves in the patient's future position, depend on many factors, and the professional team must not make superficial judgements about what appears to have been communicated to relatives or about the ways in which they are responding.

Finally, professionals also vary in their competence to understand what is at stake in the decision. In common with non-professionals, they are strongly influenced by their individual perceptions and values. They may be excessively confident that a particular outcome of treatment would be undesirable to the patient, just because it seems undesirable to them. Physicians sometimes encourage a decision to discontinue treatment because they cannot envisage valuing a life marred by disability or simply because they are ignorant of the long-term prospects for recovery and for rehabilitation. Such prejudices should be excluded from consideration. Intuition is not enough.

CONCLUSION

No single formula will resolve the complex ethical dilemmas associated with treatment decisions, but the principles enunciated here can help make the process more transparent than it could be if based solely on intuitions. The key concepts, apart from the four standard ethical principles in bioethics, are that (1) the sanctity of life is not absolute; (2) the patient is a privileged person in the medical process even though other interests should be taken into account; (3) the right people, and only the right people, should be involved in either helping the patient to reach a decision or acting on his behalf; (4) determining and respecting the patient's best interests requires not only ethical rigour but also commitment and imagination.

Acknowledgement
Thanks to Adam Zeman and Linda Emanuel for useful comments on previous drafts.

APPENDIX

The Law Commission has proposed that the following should be taken into account in assessing the best interests of the patient (Law Commission, 1995):

(1) the ascertainable past and present wishes and feelings of the person concerned, and the factors that person would consider if able to do so
(2) the need to permit and encourage the person to participate, or to improve his or her ability to participate, as fully as possible in anything done for and any decision affecting him or her
(3) the views of other people to whom it is appropriate and practicable to consult about the person's wishes and feelings and what would be in his or her best interests
(4) whether the purpose for which any action or decision is required can be as effectively achieved in a manner less restrictive of the person's freedom of action.

REFERENCES

Airdale NHS Trust v. Bland (1993) 1 All ER 821.
BMA (British Medical Association) (1992) *Rights and Responsibilities of Doctors*. London: BMA.
Bolam v. Friern Barnet Hospital Management Committee (1957) 2 All ER 118.
Bonhoeffer D (1963) *Ethics*, pp. 134–135. London: SCM Press.
Brody BA (1988) *Life and Death Decision Making*. New York: Oxford University Press.
Buchanan A and Brock D (1989) *Deciding for Others: The Ethics of Surrogate Decision Making*. Cambridge: Cambridge University Press.
Dworkin R (1977) *Taking Rights Seriously*. London: Duckworth.
F v. West Berkshire HA (1989) 2 All ER 545.
Frankfurt H (1971) Freedom of the will and the concept of a person. *Journal of Philosophy* **68**:5–20.
Gillon R (1986) *Philosophical Medical Ethics*. Chichester: John Wiley & Sons.
GMC (General Medical Council) (1995) *Duties of a Doctor*. London: GMC.
Harris J (1985) *The Value of Life: An Introduction to Medical Ethics*. London: Routledge and Kegan Paul.
Law Commission (1995) Draft Bill, clause 3 (2) quoted in McHale *et al.*, 1997, p. 305.
McHale J, Fox M and Murphy J (1997) *Health Care Law: Text and Materials*. London: Sweet & Maxwell.
McLean S (1994) *Is there a Legal Threat to Medicine?* Cardiff: Centre for Applied Ethics.
R v. Cambridge DHA, ex p. B (1995) 2 All ER 129.
Re J (A minor) (Medical treatment) (1992) 2 FLR 165.
Weir R (1989) *Abating Treatment with Critically Ill Patients: Ethical and Legal Limits to the Medical Prolongation of Life*. New York: Oxford University Press.

All ER = All England Law Reports
FLR = Family Law Reports

16

When, If Ever, Should We Expedite Death?

Diane E Meier, Hattie Myers, Phillip R Muskin

ABSTRACT

Based on a particular case, the authors review the psychological elements of responding to a patient's request for assistance in hastening death. Components considered include the patient's request as a form of communication; the problem of identifying depression in such patients and the pseudo-empathy felt by physicians for patients whose situations also seem intolerable to the doctor; physician suffering and exhaustion in the face of patient's continued suffering and the intolerance of health professionals for the feelings of helplessness; and the role of intense cost-containment pressures as they may influence the physician's ability to care for patients through long and expensive illnesses. The possible contributions of the unconscious reactions of the physician to his ill and dependent patient to a decision to assist in hastening death are reviewed.

CASE DESCRIPTION

Mrs C was a 69-year-old woman with a 10-year history of systemic lupus erythematosus. She suffered from severe osteoporosis and muscle wasting as a result of long-term corticosteroid therapy. Her collagen vascular disease manifested as progressive pulmonary disease with decreased pulmonary function and exertional dyspnoea. In spite of profound weakness, deconditioning, and musculoskeletal pain associated both with joint and skin pain and with multiple osteoporotic fractures, Mrs C continued to go to work daily at her business, though she spent increasing portions of her work day resting on a couch in the office. She lived with her husband of 45 years and had three adult children.

Mrs C was referred to Dr L, an internist with expertise in palliative care, for assistance in controlling her pain symptoms. At the initial visit, in an effort to convey the nature of her illness to the new doctor, Mrs C showed Dr L several notebooks filled with detailed notes about the 10-year course of her illness. Dr L began several pharmacological agents for treatment of pain, fatigue, and diminished nutritional status, with some success in terms of improved pain and energy levels.

In the final year of her life, as her functional capacity progressively narrowed, she began to speak to Dr L about wanting access to assistance with the timing of her death. When asked why she wanted to do this, she responded that her life was becoming too burdensome, that needing help from others for the simplest activities was unacceptable to her, and that the inability to swallow, to move without exhaustion and discomfort, was becoming unbearable. In further discussion about her life, she described her childhood. She had been adopted from an orphanage at the age of 5 years. Dependency for bathing and toileting now evoked the terror, shame, and loneliness of the orphanage for her, greatly increasing the suffering associated with her progressive decline in functional capacity. The percutaneous gastrostomy tube that she had reluctantly agreed to when her weight loss became severe was causing acid leakage onto the abdominal wall, oesophageal reflux and associated severe pain and distress. Though removing the tube was offered as an alternative by Dr L, the patient was also distressed by her marked weight loss and cachexia, and opted to maintain the tube at a lower feeding rate rather than remove it at that juncture. She could no longer sit up to read or watch television and was too weak to write. Getting to the bathroom was a major ordeal. A passionate gardener, she could no longer participate in any of her hobbies. She expressed concern about the burden that her care posed for her husband, although there were no financial problems affecting her care. Finally, she said simply 'I'm exhausted and I've had enough'. Subsequently she became too weak to get into the office and began to spend her days in bed, arising only to go to the bathroom.

Dr L responded by asking her permission to obtain a psychiatric consultation to help in the evaluation of depression. He initiated treatment with a psychostimulant, as well as a selective serotonin reuptake inhibitor. Existing doses of morphine, begun for pain and dyspnoea, were increased in an effort to relieve her feelings of 'total body aching'. To be sure that all possible treatments for the collagen vascular disease had been tried, her physician encouraged her to seek another opinion at another centre. She reluctantly agreed, saying to her husband that she was just doing it out of concern for the physician. The new rheumatologist suggested intermittent high-dose steroid infusions in the hospital. Having had long and unhappy experience with hospitals, Mrs C refused this treatment. When encouraged that it was worth a try, she agreed on the condition that, if the treatment failed and she continued to deteriorate further, she could expect help in committing suicide.

Her physician sought a second psychiatric opinion at this point. After lengthy consultations, both psychiatrists agreed that the patient was not clinically depressed. The patient remained adamant in her refusal to enter the hospital for treatment in the absence of a commitment from her physician for an 'escape route', as she called the prescription for the barbiturates recommended by Derek Humphrey's book *Final Exit* (Humphrey, 1991). The patient's husband supported her decision, purchasing *Final Exit* for her at her insistence, and helping her try to locate pills in their home that might be sufficient. The physician considered but rejected the option of telling the patient that it was in her power to stop eating and drinking at any time, thus influencing the timing of her death in a manner entirely under her own control. Dr L did not raise this possibility because he was afraid that it might be understood by her as a statement of advocacy for her hastened death. Similarly, he felt that promising her that she could be sedated to unconsciousness while foregoing food and fluids would be experienced by her as an offensive and inadequate response to her request, precisely because it did not afford her the kind of control over the timing and circumstances of her own death that she was so forcefully seeking. After discussions with colleagues and much deliberation and uncertainty, he gave her a prescription for a barbiturate with the proviso that she would not take it without first trying the steroid infusion therapy and discussing her decision in advance of any action with her husband and doctor. She agreed.

After several admissions for steroid infusions, Mrs C was no better. Her weakness was markedly worse and she could no longer make it to the bathroom. She removed her feeding tube herself because the acid burning and reflux was too painful. She continued to allow her husband to help her eat and drink small amounts at their meal-times. She had two episodes of hypnogogic hallucinations, which were frightening to her, and experienced continuous myoclonus and tremor. Adjustments in opioid dosage, rotation of opioids, addition of haloperidol and benzodiazepines, and tapering of the psychostimulant and antidepressant failed to relieve her suffering.

She described her existence as a continuous battle with her body, with drug side-effects, and with physical discomfort. She allowed a home aide to help her with personal care for the last several weeks of her life. Several days before her death, she called her children to see her and told them that she was going to die soon, implying but not explicitly stating that she was planning to commit suicide. They said good-bye to her. The next day she telephoned her husband at work as well as Dr L and said that she could not take any more, was feeling desperate, and needed help on that day. She was not willing to negotiate further. She said she feared abandonment by her doctor just when she most needed help. 'You're not going to abandon me now are you?' She expressed anger that she had been made to wait so long before being helped to die. When asked, she refused to wait until Dr L could get to the house. Her husband came home and tried to prepare the barbiturates for Mrs C. She was unable to swallow without great difficulty because of her underlying disease, so he crushed the barbiturates in ice cream and fed all 30 tablets to her. By the time the doctor arrived, Mrs C was deeply asleep, breathing 4–6 times per minute. An hour later she died.

The bereavement period was complicated by a lengthy period of major depression in the patient's husband. He had never said good-bye to her because she was so anxious and agitated at the last that he felt it impossible to try. This failure to say good-bye troubled him deeply. He suffered frequent flashbacks of feeding her the pills and often wondered aloud if she would still be here if he hadn't helped her. Three years after her death, her husband remains emotionally labile and tearful, expressing loneliness and a sense of meaninglessness during conversations with Dr L, with whom he maintains close and regular contact. In spite of regular psychotherapy and antidepressants, he has not been able to retrieve a sense of joy in life and often wonders aloud about the point of going on. Dr L still speaks to his colleagues about this case, expressing concern about whether he had done the right thing, about the unexpected and devastating consequences of this suicide for the patient's husband, and wonders what he could or should have done differently to avoid this outcome.

INTRODUCTION

A fundamental purpose of the practice of medicine is to help people through serious illness with as little distress and suffering as possible. In part as a result of the dramatic successes of modern medicine in curing disease and prolonging life, some have come to view medical care as a likely source of suffering or prolongation of suffering, rather than as a dependable source of relief. Multiple studies demonstrate inadequate treatment of pain, particularly in underserved or marginalized populations (the elderly, women, ethnic minorities, patients with HIV infection) (Cleeland, 1994; Breitbart *et al.*, 1996a,b; Cleeland *et al.*, 1997), widespread failure to identify and treat depression in the medically ill (Ganzini and Lee, 1997), and poor communication between doctor and patient regarding decisions near the end of life (SUPPORT Principal Investigators, 1995). These inadequacies persist despite repeated exhortations from professional societies and in the medical literature. Perhaps in part as a response to witnessing these experiences and not trusting the medical profession to relieve suffering and respect patients' wishes, public opinion polls consistently suggest that a majority of respondents favour legalization of physician-assisted death under circumstances of intolerable suffering near the end of life (Meier *et al.*, 1998). The state of Oregon in the United States (Oregon Death with Dignity Act, 1995) and the Northern Territory of Australia (Ryan and Kaye, 1996) have been the first to legalize access to a doctor's aid in dying, and similar efforts are underway in other locations.

In spite of the growing support from the general public, professional medical organizations remain largely opposed to the legalization of physician-assisted suicide. Practising physicians are divided in their views, with surveys of physicians demonstrating from 30–60% of respondents in favour of legalization under carefully defined circumstances (Meier *et al.*, 1998). Recent surveys of physicians in the United States suggest that physician-assisted death remains rare: about 6% of doctors in specialties closely involved with the care of dying patients report having had at least one such experience (with a median of two) in their practice lifetime (Meier *et al.*, 1998). However, this study also showed that a substantially higher proportion, 18.3%, had received at least one request from a patient for assistance in dying, suggesting that education is needed to prepare physicians to respond appropriately to such requests.

Legalization of physician-assisted suicide might also have a substantial impact on a physician's willingness to assist in a patient's death. In the same study (Meier *et al.*, 1998), willingness to participate in physician-assisted death tripled from 11 to 36% if laws were changed to permit it. A substantial proportion of Dutch physicians now have either directly participated in assisting a patient to die, or favour continued access to the option (van der Maas *et al.*, 1996). Thus, there is reason to believe that the practice would become significantly more common under circumstances where it was legal to do so. Guidelines have been proposed to safeguard patients from coercion, involuntary euthanasia, or unrecognized/untreated depression (Quill *et al.*, 1992), and different versions are currently employed in Oregon and Australia. But the issue of exploring both the patient's and the physician's motivations, conscious and unconscious, when responding to this type of request has not been addressed. As in the case described here, the patient's motives are often complex and not readily apparent unless carefully and skillfully sought.

The patient–physician relationship in the context of care for a very sick or dying patient is, by its fundamentally dependent and imbalanced nature, informed by powerful emotional connections, sometimes conscious but often unconscious. Heightened awareness of these psychological forces is important both to enhance compassionate care of the dying, and also to anchor public policy deliberations in the real world of doctor and patient. In spite of the powerful psychological determinants of a request for assistance with suicide and of the physician's response to such a request, with some exceptions (Block and Billings, 1994; Miles, 1994; Muskin, 1998) most prior work on the question of physician-assisted suicide has focused on the morality and ethics of such an act, its consequences for society, and the problems of crafting public policy for such a medically and legally complex activity. Rather than revisit these aspects of the debate, in this chapter we examine the psychological aspects of the relationship between doctor and patient as it influences the process of decision-making when a patient requests a doctor's help in committing suicide.

REQUEST AS COMMUNICATION

The distinction between the manifest content of a communication from a patient and its unconscious meaning is of fundamental importance in a patient's request for a doctor's help in committing suicide. Failure to explore the possible meanings (Quill, 1993) of such a request, and failure to be aware of the physician's own complex responses to it, may lead to a patient's premature death and irrevocably missed opportunities to identify and relieve suffering, and to complete critical life tasks in the period before death. A patient's request for help in committing suicide is, first and foremost, a communication to the doctor of great distress, and it implies an expectation of some kind of response from the doctor (Muskin, 1998). Either a yes or a no response from the doctor can be a form of abandonment in this situation. A physician who responds by agreeing that the patient's continued life is intolerable, that if he were in their shoes death would indeed be preferable, sends the message that the patient's life is not of sufficient value to fight for and that the doctor can no longer bear to witness and thus share in the patient's suffering. Conversely, a physician who responds by withdrawing from his patient, suggesting that such a request is offensive or burdensome or unethical, or trivializes it with 'Don't be silly, of course you're not going to do something like that!' commits another type of abandonment by failing to heed the communication hidden in the request and by leaving his patient alone with his desperation and hopelessness. To avoid these traps, further engagement with the patient is required, manifested by a willingness to listen to the patient's distress, a commitment to explore the reasons behind the request, to sustained effort to reduce sources of suffering and search for a reason to continue, and reassurance to the patient that his physician will be there, come what may, until the end. A recent essay by Emanuel (1998) outlines a step-wise approach to patient requests for a hastened death that seeks to identify the root causes, ensures optimal palliative care, allows discontinuation of unwanted life-prolonging therapies, and requires continued engagement of patient and doctor through the course of the illness, short of providing assistance with an earlier death.

DEPRESSION AND 'PSEUDO-EMPATHY'

Evidence suggests that physicians frequently fail to identify and treat depression when it occurs in office practice as well as in the context of medical illness (Ganzini and Lee, 1997). The problem of pseudo-empathy (Sullivan and Youngner, 1993) or physician over-identification with the patient's plight, and the unexamined assumption that therefore the depression is rational, may result in undertreatment of depression and missed opportunities to restore meaning and will to live in spite of the continuing illness. This is of particular importance in the context of requests for assistance in dying since several studies have identified depression as an important predictor of suicidal thoughts in medically ill patients (Chochinov *et al.*, 1995; Breitbart *et al.*, 1996a; Emanuel *et al.*, 1996). In spite of these data, prevalence studies have shown that physician referrals to psychiatry for evaluation following a request for a hastened death are rare (Back *et al.*, 1996; Meier *et al.*, 1998), and that physician identification and diagnosis of depression in this clinical circumstance are similarly uncommon. Whether pharmacological or psychotherapeutic treatment of depression would affect the patient's wish to die is unknown and requires study, but a trial of therapy is inarguable and should be mandatory prior to considering provision of assistance with a hastened death (Emanuel, 1998). Oregon law does not require psychiatric referral in response to the request unless the referring physician thinks that a disorder affecting judgement or decisional capacity may be present (Oregon Death with Dignity Act, 1995): future safeguards should probably require psychiatric evaluation for the presence of depression as well as other, often subtle, psychiatric disorders including anxiety, delirium, and mild dementia.

A thorough psychiatric evaluation of a patient requesting assistance in committing suicide should not be conceptualized as a one-visit event leading to a definitive opinion, as occurred in the case presented here. Only 6% of Oregon psychiatrists felt they could perform an adequate evaluation in a single session (Ganzini and Lee, 1997). In addition, there is a subgroup of patients who will benefit from psychotherapy in the terminal phase of life, which may greatly reduce their suffering (Druss, 1995; Eissler, 1955). In spite of repeated evaluations and pharmacotherapy for depression, Mrs C's emotional distress in the face of her illness was not relieved. She declined on-going psychotherapy although it was offered and encouraged on several occasions.

Many of the physicians involved in her care towards the end of her life expressed pity and understanding of her wish to die. This example of a pseudo-empathy reaction of 'Of course, I would be depressed and want to die too if I were in that situation,' grows out of the physician's terror of the patient's circumstances, identification with the patient's suffering and helplessness, and the physician's sense of failure and impotence at not being able to fix it. Such a physician reaction, rather than encouraging and helping the patient in their struggle, reinforces and supports the patient's own estimation of his situation (Muskin, 1998). Physicians are often particularly intolerant of lack of power and control and particularly unwilling to accept the fact that there are some things that cannot be fixed or made better. Thus, in the case described, in spite of repeated and sophisticated efforts to relieve physical and emotional symptoms, Mrs C's suffering could not be adequately ameliorated. The lack of control over the disease and its consequences was unbearably distressing for patient and physician alike.

In this situation, Dr L's agreement to provide a prescription for barbiturates did not appear to derive from anger at Mrs C for failing to respond to treatment nor to his need to end his own suffering through her death. He considered and addressed the possibility of depression and he was aggressive in her pain and symptom management. The patient's evident misery, and her courage in the face of all that she had been through, made assisting in her suicide seem to Dr L to be the least he could do, since all other medical interventions he had tried seemed to be of limited, and diminishing, benefit. The suicide option gave Mrs C the strength to keep trying new treatments along with a sense of control over the profound helplessness occasioned by her progressive disease. A key element in this action by the physician, therefore, was his engagement, empathy, and knowledge of his patient as a person.

Continuing to refuse to accede to her request at that point was understood by the patient (and her doctor) as yet another abandonment. The patient's own terror of abandonment, her rage at her husband and doctor for failing to help her earlier, her deep aversion to dependence on others for personal care, were clearly connected to her earliest life experiences. Yet awareness of and discussion about this connection with her doctor as well as with two psychiatrists failed to change her intolerance for her situation. Similarly, awareness of the psychological roots of much of her suffering did not reduce the pressure her physician felt to honour her request. The existence of the bottle of pills which had earlier allowed pursuit of further medical interventions, now seemed to close discussion of all other avenues, including the option of foregoing food and water. Both the patient's need for control over the rapid downward spiral of events and her physician's need to be responsive to her request for help led to an assisted suicide.

This phenomenon of intolerance for helplessness on the part of both patient and physician has implications for the legalization of assisted suicide. Physicians' inability to live with this reality may create empathy and support for the patients' conclusion that continued life under the burden imposed by the illness is intolerable. Thus an expression of despair becomes a fixed belief that no alternative but suicide is possible, a position unconsciously aided and abetted by the physician's sympathy for the patient's suicidal plans, and fuelled by the physician's suffering. 'After all', the patient may reason, 'even my doctor, who is supposed to be on my side and should be the strongest advocate for my continued life, agrees with me that I'm better off dead.' The patient's action in pursuing suicide may then be seen in part as an attempt to relieve the *physician's* suffering or even as an angry response to the physician's advocacy for, instead of opposition to, her death (Muskin, 1998). In the case described here, Dr L's advocacy for Mrs C's death, as expressed by provision of the prescription, may have been experienced as a re-enactment of her earliest abandonment during infancy. These powerful emotions, often unconscious in both patient and physician, may heighten pressures towards premature closure through expediting the patient's death.

Physicians' feelings of helplessness and lack of tolerance for feeling helpless are inextricably linked to a decision to assist a patient to die but do not provide a rational or ethical basis for such an act. In no existing policy regarding assisted suicide are there provisions for examination of the unconscious motivations of the physician. The need for education to assist physicians to understand their own reactions to the care of a terminally ill patient is not likely to become a routine part of medical training, nor is such a process mandated in any policy legalizing physician-assisted suicide. Given these constraints, Miles wrote, 'Public policy with respect to legalization of physician assisted suicide must respect and recognize these forces and act to protect patients from them' (Miles, 1995).

The impact on families and survivors of a patient who dies by suicide is not well understood but, as suggested by the case described here, the risk of complicated bereavement seems to be greater following a death by suicide (Saunders and Sykes, 1993). Whether this phenomenon differs among family survivors of patients in terminal stages who hasten death by relatively short periods is unknown and deserves study, but the consequences for family may be severe and longlasting. There is an ancient Chinese proverb that suggests that a suicide reverberates for seven generations. In this context, the principle of autonomy upon which a public policy of legal physician-assisted suicide is based does little to inform the calculus of competing emotional, physical, and material needs and pressures surrounding a seriously ill patient and her family and professional caregivers.

PROFESSIONAL SUFFERING

A physician's sense of helplessness and frustration in the face of chronic, progressive, and devastating illness may lead to an unconscious advocacy for suicide as the best means of controlling the uncontrollable, and eliminating the strain and distress of the illness for patient and doctor alike (Miles, 1994, 1995; Muskin, 1998). The training of modern physicians, and perhaps the self-selection process involved in choosing the medical profession, instills a sense of control that allows physicians to believe that all disease can and should be successfully mastered and managed. Even among palliative care experts where there is a recognition that death is inevitable, there is a belief that all, or the vast majority, of suffering can be relieved (Foley, 1991). While this may be true in most cases, there remain some individuals who continue to suffer intolerably in spite of access to good palliative care. Such situations present a similarly intolerable conflict for physicians whose role is therefore reduced to witnessing this suffering with associated feelings of loss of control and powerlessness to help.

The difficulty of attending to a suffering and dying person, particularly when repeated efforts to provide relief have been ineffective, often leads to a sense of professional failure, guilt, frustration, and exhaustion. Unconscious feelings of irritation and anger may also accompany the care of difficult, demanding, and time-intensive patients. Many physicians respond to the dread and demoralization that accompanies this stage of disease by withdrawal, visiting less, spending less time at each visit, and letting others provide the day-to-day care. Agreeing with the patient that suicide is a rational option can be another form of this type of abandonment (Block and Billings, 1994; Miles, 1994, 1995; Muskin, 1998). The patient may detect this and accede to his doctor's wish by ending his life.

The power of the physician in the sick patient's life also has important similarities to that of a parent to his child. The physician is imbued with omnipotent powers and symbolizes the loving parent, advocating forcefully for his patient's life and health (Muskin, 1998). When the doctor/parent gives up and is no longer able to tolerate the pain of caring for the patient, the sick person's already vulnerable sense of worth and value is further threatened. Understanding the profound symbolic power of the physician in relation to his patient is critical to maintaining a healing stance, even in the face of continued suffering and distress, and underscores the importance of a consistent advocacy for the value of the patient's continued life. Agreeing to assist a patient to commit suicide should not be undertaken without an awareness of the depth of influence over the patient that this agreement inevitably carries.

Physicians are not well trained to reflect upon and analyse the feelings of distress and helplessness precipitated by caring for a dying patient nor with a sick patient's request for help with suicide. Further, physicians are not trained to find personal and professional meaning and satisfaction in caring, sometimes for a very long time, for a patient who is suffering and dying despite their best efforts and who, further, is struggling to find their own meaning in the process. It is emotionally demanding, often emotionally consuming, to remain intimate and responsive in the face of uncertainty and ambiguity as patients sicken, suffer, and come near to death. Rather, physicians are trained to find meaning and satisfaction in the 'saves', those patients who do well, get better and go, gratefully, home. Given the forces arrayed against doctors' ability to stand with their patients as they suffer and die, it may not be possible to ensure a level of psychological sophistication in physicians sufficient to prevent unwitting advocacy for suicide as the 'best of a bunch of bad options'. As Miles argues, the presence of a taboo against physician-assisted suicide may serve as a needed check in the demanding process of care for a dying patient in great emotional distress (Miles, 1994). Given the temptation that legal-assisted suicide presents to exhausted doctors, families and patients, and given the degree of psychological dependency of a very ill patient, the potential for subtle and unintentional complicity and influence should assisted suicide become widely legal, is troubling, and suggests that legalization is, at best, premature.

COST PRESSURES ON MEDICAL CARE FOR THE TERMINALLY ILL

The overwhelming cost-containment forces now characterizing the practice of medicine in the United States are increasingly relevant to this debate. Physician payment incentives accompanying managed care and capitated plans financially reward providing less medical care for the patient (Meier, 1997). The burden of diminished access to needed resources (such as prescription medicines, home care attendants, hospitalization) falls not only on the patient, but importantly on the physician (who cannot meet all of the dying patient's medical needs alone, but has ever-diminished access to other professional resources), and most powerfully on the patient's family who must pay in both time and resources for whatever is not provided by the health care system (SUPPORT Principal Investigators, 1995). In the context of highly labour- and technology-intensive terminal illnesses, the temptation to patient, family and doctor to solve these tensions through resort to an expedited death is obvious. This combination of forces—emotional and physical dependency of seriously ill patients on family and doctor, economic constraints on needed resources, physical and mental exhaustion of patient and caregivers, the subtle but powerful psychological issues inevitable in these demanding relationships, all combined with the societal advocacy that legalization would represent for physician-assisted death—makes the concept of a truly autonomous patient choice seem highly idealistic. To the extent that a public policy legalizing physician-assisted death is based on the assumption of genuine patient autonomy, these interdependent and complex relational and economic issues between the patient, family, and doctor suggest that true patient autonomy under such circumstances is unlikely.

CONCLUSION

When, if ever, should a patient's death be expedited? A patient's request for assistance in dying is a signal of great distress. Sometimes this distress can be adequately relieved through symptom management, psychotherapy, and spiritual and psychosocial support. Negotiated discontinuation of life-sustaining therapies, including food and fluid, combined with analgesia and sedation necessary to relieve suffering, may be an acceptable alternative to most patients seeking a hastened death (Emanuel, 1998). Such an approach should be advocated in place of physician-assisted suicide. Sometimes, however, such options are unacceptable or inadequate responses to a patient's evaluation of his or her own needs and desires as they are dying, as in the case presented here. The prohibition on physician-assisted suicide should not be an excuse to disengage from the suffering patient, just as legalization should not be an excuse to avoid the difficult process of understanding the reason for the request and trying to help the patient find a reason to go on. There are rare patients for whom no other course is acceptable and the physician feels that he must either accede to the patient's request or effectively abandon the patient to suffer. Such a decision is inevitably and irreducibly influenced by the doctor's desire to bring his or her own sense of helplessness and discomfort to a close as well (Miles, 1994). Awareness of this fact is critical to avoid unintentional coercion and influence when dying patients face their few remaining choices.

Jecker wrote that 'care for another may make it morally impossible to simply step aside and watch a protracted illness run its course' (Jecker, 1991). Though the case described here, and others like it, provide compelling support for Jecker's assertion, they do not provide a sound and principled basis for a public policy permitting physician-assisted suicide. The potential for subtle coercion of the seriously ill is real: not only does our society fail to provide adequate insurance coverage for the medical needs of large numbers of the terminally ill and their exhausted and overburdened family members, but the fact of legalization in and of itself is coercive as we no longer promote the value of each life and instead sanction an expedient death rather than take on the costs of continued care and support. When combined with the complex transference issues attending every patient–physician and family–patient relationship, it seems clear that legalization poses a risk to vulnerable persons with terminal illness. Maintaining laws against physician-assisted suicide means that some patients will not receive assistance in dying that might otherwise have seemed right and proper. But no policy can meet all needs and public policy must serve the greatest good.

Enhanced awareness of the psychological pressures on physicians whose patients request assistance in suicide, combined with a commitment to stand by the patient with provision of ongoing care and support may help physicians to have the fortitude to help their patients through this most difficult of times. Thus, we advocate managing suffering in all of its dimensions—physical, emotional, and interpersonal, spiritual, and social—and we have identified reason to pause before advocating expediting a death as the best available intervention. At the individual level, premature positions on actions that may cause strong and unpredictable emotions in any of the key parties can foreclose effective therapeutic encounters and decisions. The physician's steady attempts to relieve suffering must be accompanied by the maintenance of the patient–physician relationship until the final moment of life. This creates a tension essential to the balance between the physician's obligation to preserve life and the sometimes countervailing obligation to relieve suffering.

As in many aspects of life the Bible may provide some guidance in this issue (for this particular insight we thank Rabbi Kenneth A Stern; Stern, 1998). As Abraham raises his knife to sacrifice his son Isaac (Genesis 22:10), does he know he will be stopped? In that moment, his hand raised, the muscles tensed to bring down the knife, Abraham must live through his suffering as he proceeds with what he believes he must do, according to his faith. Although patients are not our children, powerful emotions nonetheless link physicians and patients, especially as the physician witnesses sometimes extreme periods of suffering and as they approach together the moment of the patient's death. We might then take this message from the Bible: no moment is over until it has passed irrevocably. Expediting death will always bring premature closure because the patient, physician, or both will have elected not to live through the person's life until the end. This is never true of the devotion to alleviate suffering—each moment is lived, by patient and physician, until it has passed. Some may observe that this approach is too difficult, too painful, too filled with uncertainty for 'modern medicine'. It is exactly such powerful emotions that will protect the integrity and depth of medical care wherever technology or legislation may lead us.

REFERENCES

Back AI, Wallace JI, Starks HE and Pearlman RA (1996) Physician assisted suicide and euthanasia in Washington State. *Journal of the American Medical Association* **275**:919–925.

Block SD and Billings JA (1994) Patient requests to hasten death. *Archives of Internal Medicine* **154**:2039–2047.

Breitbart W, Rosenfeld BD and Passik SD (1996a) Interest in physician-assisted suicide among ambulatory HIV-infected patients. *American Journal of Psychiatry* **153**:238–242.

Breitbart W, Rosenfeld BD, Passik SD *et al.* (1996b) The undertreatment of pain in ambulatory AIDS patients. *Pain* **65**:243–249.

Chochinov HM, Wilson KG, Enns M *et al.* (1995) Desire for death in the terminally ill. *American Journal of Psychiatry* **152**:1185–1191.

Cleeland CS (1994) Pain and its treatment in outpatients with metastatic cancer. *New England Journal of Medicine* **330**:592–596.

Cleeland CS, Gonin K, Baez L *et al.* (1997) Pain and treatment of pain in minority patients with cancer. *Annals of Internal Medicine* **127**:813–816.

Druss RG (1995) *The Psychology of Illness*. Washington, DC:American Psychiatric Press.

Eissler KR (1955) *The Psychiatrist and the Dying Patient*. New York, New York: International Universities Press.

Emanuel EJ, Fairclough DL, Daniels ER and Clarridge BR (1996) Euthanasia and physician-assisted suicide: Attitudes and experiences of oncology patients, oncologists, and the public. *Lancet* **347**:1805–1810.

Emanuel LL (1998) Facing requests for physician-assisted suicide: Toward a practical and principled clinical skill set. *Journal of the American Medical Association* **280**:643–647.

Foley KM (1991) The relationship of pain and symptom management to patient requests for physician-assisted suicide. *Journal of Pain and Symptom Management* **6**:289–297.

Ganzini L and Lee M (1997) Psychiatry and assisted suicide in the United States. *New England Journal of Medicine* **336**:1823–1826.

Humphrey D (1991) *Final Exit: The Practicalities of Self-Deliverance and Assisted Suicide For the Dying*. Eugene, Oregon: Hemlock Society.

Jecker NS (1991) Giving death a hand: When the dying and the doctor stand in a special relationship. *Journal of the American Geriatrics Society* **39**:831–835.

Meier DE (1997) Voiceless and vulnerable: Dementia patients without surrogates in an era of capitation. *Journal of the American Geriatrics Society* **45**:375–377.

Meier DE, Emmons CA, Wallenstein S *et al.* (1998) A national survey of physician-assisted death and euthanasia in the United States. *New England Journal of Medicine* **338**:1193–1201.

Miles SH (1994) Physicians and their patients' suicides. *Journal of the American Medical Association* **271**:1786–1788.

Miles SH (1995) Physician assisted suicide and the profession's gyrocompass. *Hastings Center Report* **25**:17–19.

Muskin PR (1998) The request to die: Role for a psychodynamic perspective on physician-assisted suicide. *Journal of the American Medical Association* **279**:323–328.

Oregon Death with Dignity Act (1995) Or Laws Ch. 3 (initiative measure No. 16).

Quill TE (1993) Doctor, I want to die. Will you help me? *Journal of the American Medical Association* **270(7)**:870–873.

Quill TE, Cassel CK and Meier DE (1992) Care of the hopelessly ill: Proposed clinical criteria for physician-assisted suicide. *New England Journal of Medicine* **327**:1380–1384.

Ryan CJ and Kaye M (1996) Euthanasia in Australia—The Northern Territory Rights of the Terminally Ill Act. *New England Journal of Medicine* **334**:326–328.

Saunders C and Sykes N (1993) *The Management of Terminal Disease*, 3rd edn. London: Edward Arnold.

Stern, Rabbi Kenneth (1998) Sermon, Park Avenue Synagogue, New York, NY.

Sullivan MD and Youngner SJ (1993) Depression, competence, and the right to refuse lifesaving medical treatment. *American Journal of Psychiatry* **151**:971–978.

SUPPORT Principal Investigators (1995) A controlled trial to improve care for seriously ill hospitalized patients. *Journal of the American Medical Association* **274**:591–598.

van der Maas PJ, van der Wal G, Haverkate I *et al.* (1996) Euthanasia, physician-assisted suicide, and other medical practices involving the end of life in the Netherlands, 1990–1995. *New England Journal of Medicine* **335**:1699–1705.

17

Is the Concept of Brain Death Secure?

Calixto Machado

ABSTRACT

Any full account of death should include three distinct elements: a definition of death, its anatomical substratum, and the tests required to diagnose it. The three main brain-oriented formulations of death are the 'whole brain', the 'brainstem' and the 'higher brain' standards. This essay outlines and criticize these accounts, proposing a new standard of human death based on the physiological mechanisms of consciousness generation. Consciousness has two physiological components: arousal and awareness. As brainstem-diencephalic and cortical structures interact to generate consciousness, any rigid distinction between functions their would be misleading. Substantial interconnections among the brainstem, subcortical structures and the neocortex serve both components of human consciousness. Therefore, consciousness generation is based on anatomy and physiology throughout the brain. None of the three current brain-oriented formulations is wholly satisfactory. The proposed standard of human death identifies consciousness as the most important function of the body, because it provides the key human attribute and the highest level of control in the hierarchy of integrating functions within the human organism.

INTRODUCTION

Since ancient times, man has pondered the mystery of death. In discovering the meaning of death, he hoped to find the explanation of life (Machado, 1995, pp. V–VI). In the earliest records, life was held to continue as long as an individual breathed. It was later thought that respiration was a means of maintaining the heart that circulated the blood. Life was then attributed to cardiorespiratory action. But, in the middle of this century, physicians became aware that the brain required much more energy than other organs. If the brain's needs were not met it would cease to function, while other parts of the body could remain viable and even regain their activity, provided that respiration and circulation were maintained by artificial substitution in intensive care units (Walker, 1981; Pernick, 1988; Machado *et al.*, 1995). This was documented by French neurologists and neurophysiologists at the end of the 1950s (Mollaret and Goulon, 1995; Wertheimer *et al.*, 1959) The result would be a dead brain in a viable body. Is such a 'preparation' alive or dead? (Walker, 1981).

The end of the 1960s brought further prominent advances in this area. The Ad Hoc Committee of Harvard Medical School proposed, for the first time, a new neurological criterion of death (Beecher, 1968). Harvard's report appeared some months after Christian Barnard's first transplantation of a human heart, in December of 1967.

The 1980s and the 1990s have been characterized by multidisciplinary debates. In 1981 the President's Commission for the Study of Ethical Problems in Medicine and Behavioral Research issued a report on defining death (Guidelines, 1981; President's Commission). There are still world-wide controversies over the neurological definition of death: should it require death of the whole brain, the brainstem or the neocortex? There is also disagreement about how to diagnose brain death, whether by clinical means alone, or with the help of ancillary tests (Machado *et al.*, 1995). Moreover, a group of scholars who were strong defenders of a brain-based standard of death are now favoring a circulatory-respiratory view (Shewmon, 1997; Truog, 1997; Shewmon, 1998a,b).

Any full account of death should include three distinct elements: the definition of death, the criterion (anatomical substratum) of brain death, and the tests to prove that the criterion has been satisfied (Bernat, 1981, 1984; Bartlett and Youngner, 1988; Bernat, 1991, 1992a, b; Halery and Brody, 1993; Bernat, 1998). Undoubtedly, the term 'criterion' for referring to the anatomical substratum introduces confusion in this discussion, because protocols of tests (clinical and instrumental) for brain diagnosis are called 'diagnostic criteria' or 'sets of diagnostic criteria'. Therefore, the term 'anatomical substratum' replaces criterion in this essay.

Three main brain-oriented formulations of death have been described historically: whole brain, brainstem and higher brain standards (Machado 1994, 1995, pp. V–VI, 57–66).

The whole brain standard refers to the irreversible cessation of all intracranial structure functions (Beecher, 1968; Korein, 1977; Walker, 1977; Molinari, 1980; Bernat, 1981; Guidelines, 1981; President's Commission, 1981; Bernat, 1984, 1991, 1999). Until recently, proponents of the whole brain standard had not provided a conceptual background to support specific anatomical substrata and tests (Beecher, 1968; Walker, 1977; Molinari, 1980; Walker, 1981). Moreover, this view has not specified the critical quantity and location of neurones which subserve the essential brain activities that integrate the functioning of the organism (Deliyannakis *et al.*, 1975; Ashwal and Schneider, 1979; Ferbert *et al.*, 1986; Fiser *et al.*, 1987; Howlett *et al.*, 1989; Truog, 1997).

The brainstem standard was adopted in several Commonwealth countries (Conference of Royal Colleges, 1976, 1979; Jennett, 1981; Jennett and Hessett,

1981). This view has been powerfully articulated by Christopher Pallis (Pallis and Maggillivray, 1980; Pallis, 1983a; Pallis and Prior, 1983; Pallis, 1989, 1990a). Pallis emphasized that the capacity for consciousness and respiration are the two hallmarks of life of the human being, and that brainstem death predicts an inescapable asystole (Pallis, 1990a). However, a pathophysiological review of consciousness generation will provide a basis for not accepting Pallis' definition of death (Machado, 1994, 1995, pp. 57–66). Moreover, recent clinical cases have shown that brain death does not always predict an 'inevitable asystole within a short while' (Shewmon, 1997, 1998a).

The higher brain formulation springs largely from consideration of the persistent vegetative state (PVS), and has been mainly defended by philosophers (Machado, 1994). The higher brain theorists have defined human death as the 'the loss of consciousness' (definition), related to the irreversible destruction of the neocortex (anatomical substratum) (Veatch, 1972, 1977; Green and Wikler, 1980; Bartlett and Youngner, 1988; Veatch, 1989; Cranford and Smith, 1990; Truog and Flacker, 1992).

This essay demonstrates that consciousness does not bear a simple one-to-one relationship with higher or lower brain structures and that the higher brain formation is wrong, because the definition (consciousness) does not harmonize with the anatomical substratum (neocortex). It discusses key aspects of the three brain-oriented formulations, and proposes a new standard of human death, based on the pathophysiological mechanisms of consciousness generation (Machado, 1994, 1995, pp. 57–66).

MECHANISMS OF CONSCIOUSNESS GENERATION

Plum and Posner (1980) proposed that consciousness is 'the state of awareness of self and the environment'. According to these authors, consciousness has two physiological components: arousal and awareness. Arousal is also known as capacity for consciousness (Pallis and Maggillivray, 1980; Pallis, 1983a; Pallis and Prior, 1983; Pallis, 1989, 1990a). It describes the group of behavioural changes that occurs when a person awakens from sleep or transits to a state of alertness (Moruzzi and Magoun, 1949; Plum and Posner, 1980; Plum, 1991; Kinney and Samuels, 1994; Multi-Society Task Force, 1994; Machado, 1995, pp. 57–66; Steriade, 1996). The most easily recognized of these changes is eye opening (Plum and Posner, 1980; Kirney and Samuels, 1994; Machado, 1995, pp. 57–66). These changes are particularly dependent upon the function of upper brainstem, thalamus and posterior hypothalamus, through a neuronal network known as the ascending reticular activating system (ARAS) (Moruzzi and Magoun, 1949). Awareness, also known as content of consciousness, denotes the sum of cognitive and affective mental functions and provides the knowledge of one's existence, and the conscious perception of the internal and external worlds (Plum and Posner, 1980; Machado, 1995, pp. 57–66). In summary, a human being's state of consciousness reflects his or her level of arousal, which depends on subcortical arousal-energizing systems and the sum of the cognitive, affective, and other higher brain functions (Plum and Posner, 1980; Machado, 1995, pp. 57–66). Therefore, in this essay the term 'arousal' refers to those subcortical arousal-energizing systems, and 'awareness' denotes the sum of those complex brain functions related to limbic and cerebrum levels (Machado, 1995, pp. 57–66).

Unfortunately, there are some misunderstandings when the term consciousness is used. Most authors (Veatch, 1977; Bartlett and Youngner, 1988; Truog and Flacker, 1992) mention consciousness without considering its two components, originally described by Plum and Posner (1980). For example, defenders of the higher brain theory usually describe patients in the persistent vegetative state (PVS) as having 'irreversible loss of consciousness' or being 'permanently unconscious', but in these cases arousal is preserved while awareness is apparently lost (Veatch, 1972, 1977; Green and Wikler, 1980; Bartlett and Youngner, 1988; Veatch, 1989; Cranford and Smith, 1990; Truog Flacker, 1992). Moreover, some authors mention the higher brain criterion as 'the irreversible loss of the capacity for consciousness', but they are really referring to awareness (Truog and Flacker, 1992). Considering that the use of the term 'capacity for consciousness' (Pallis and Maggillivray, 1980; Pallis and Prior, 1983; Pallis, 1989, 1990a) could be confusing, this essay uses the original term, i.e. arousal to denote the function; and awareness as a synonym for content of consciousness (Machado, 1994, 1995, pp. 57–66).

It has been argued that brainstem-diencephalic and cortical structures interact to generate consciousness, so any rigid distinction between their functions, in terms of arousal and awareness, would be misleading (Plum, 1991; Kinney and Samuels, 1994; Multi-Society Task Force, 1994; Machodo, 1995, pp. 57–66). For instance, bilateral thalamic infarcts are commonly accompanied by mental impairment, such as dementia and amnesia (Guberman and Stuss, 1983). Thus, we cannot simply differentiate and locate arousal as a function of the ARAS, and awareness as a function of the cerebral cortex. Substantial interconnections among the brainstem, subcortical structures and the neocortex, are essential for subserving and integrating both components of human consciousness (Machado, 1994, 1995, pp. 57–66).

BRAIN ANATOMY ORIENTED STANDARDS OF DEATH

Some representative clinical cases can introduce the discussion about the three main standards of death on neurological grounds.

THE WHOLE BRAIN STANDARD

Case A

The patient (JA) was 36 years old. He suffered an accident when driving his motorcycle. On arrival at the emergency room, he was deeply comatose with wide pupils, absent eye movements, and absent brainstem reflexes. He was in respiratory arrest, but had preserved cardiac function. He was immediately intubated for ventilatory assistance. Computer tomography (CT) scan showed acute hydrocephalus, and an electroencephalogram (EEG) taken during this phase did not reveal any electrical activity. A second EEG was done, applying a higher sensitivity of $2\,\mu V$ per division, and delta activity was undoubtedly recorded during 5 days. Afterwards, the EEG remained isoelectric for the rest of his clinical evolution (10 days). A test battery of multimodality evoked potentials (MEP) and electroretinography (ERG) were applied to this patient. Brainstem auditory evoked potentials showed bilateral preservation of wave I. Short latency somatosensory evoked responses consisted in the absence of the lemniscal and cortical components and preservation of the brachial plexus and spinal waves. A normal electroretinogram was recorded; meanwhile visual evoked responses were absent. He did not suffer from diabetes insipidus, and several tests showed persistence of hypothalamic neuroendocrine functions. Is this patient alive or dead?

James Bernat and his collaborators have presented the most complete defence of this standard (Bernat, 1981; Bernat *et al.*, 1981; Bernat *et al.*, 1982; Bernat, 1984; Bernat *et al.*, 1984).

Definition
The permanent cessation of the functioning of the organism as a whole.

Early whole brain defenders (Beecher, 1968; Walker, 1977; Molinari, 1980; Walker, 1981) had not provided a conceptual framework to support this criterion until Bernat and his collaborators fully elaborated this formulation. These authors defined death as 'the permanent cessation of the functioning of the organism as a whole'. By 'organism as a whole' they were not referring to the 'whole organism', as a sum of its parts, 'but rather to that characteristic that makes the living organism greater than the sum of its parts'. Furthermore, Bernat (1991) illustrated his conception of integration as follows: 'functions of the organism as a whole include respiration, temperature control, fluid and electrolyte homeostasis, consciousness, food-seeking behavior, sexual behavior, neuroendocrine regulation, and autonomic control'. Bernat (1991, 1992) postulated that the 'organism as a whole' could be still functioning, despite destruction of some subsystems.

Anatomical substratum
The permanent cessation of the functioning of the entire brain.

The anatomical substratum of this view refers to the irreversible cessation of function in all intracranial structures.

Tests
Bernat (1991) proposed two sets of tests: the permanent absence of breathing and heartbeat, and brain cessation tests. The cardiorespiratory tests are used to show the permanent loss of all brain functions, because a sustained arrest of circulation or respiration will produce ischaemia, anoxia and subsequent necrosis of the brain. The cardiorespiratory tests are applied 'in all cases except when death needs to be declared in a patient with heartbeat on a ventilator'. Hence, 'brain death tests are necessary only for patients being mechanically ventilated'. These sets of criteria included a group of preconditions and a battery of tests and clinical procedures performed at the bedside. Periods of

observation are required to carry out a second examination, in order to demonstrate the permanent absence of brain functions.

Critique

Case A illustrates the difficulties in applying this definition of neurological death. Several authors have described patients as 'whole brain dead' and yet expressed surprise when they find that the EEG is retained. The persistence of EEG activity is indeed incompatible with the diagnosis of 'whole brain death' (Deliyannakis *et al*, 1975; Ashwal and Schneider, 1979). The persistence of hypothalamic neuroendocrine functions in otherwise 'whole brain dead' patients is likewise difficult to reconcile with 'whole brain death' (Outwater and Rockoff, 1984; Fiser *et al.*, 1987; Howlett *et al.*, 1989; Hagl *et al.*, 1997; Lugo *et al.*, 1997).

These difficulties point to an underlying flaw in the 'whole brain' acount of death: it fails to specify the critical number and location of neurones required to subserve the essential activities of the hemispheres, diencephalon and brainstem, and thereby to execute the functions of the 'organism as a whole'.

THE BRAINSTEM STANDARD

Case B

FC was a 48-year-old male who suddenly lost consciousness while watching TV with his family. On arrival at the emergency room he was deeply comatose with pinpoint pupils, absent eye movements, and absent corneal reflexes, but preserved gag, cough, and breathing. He was intubated initially for airway protection. By 12 hours after admission there was no spontaneous breathing, the pupils were 4 mm and non-reactive, and all brainstem reflexes were gone. Repeat CT showed a massive brainstem haemorrhage, complicated by acute hydrocephalus due to obliteration of the IVth ventricle; however intracranial pressure was only 15 mmHg. Blood flow (by radionuclide angiogram) appeared good in the cerebral hemispheres. EEG looked like a stage II sleep record (there were even some spindles), but did not react to external stimuli. A test battery conformed by multimodality evoked potentials (MEP) and electroretinography (ERG) was applied to this patient. Brainstem auditory evoked potentials showed no response. Short latency somatosensory evoked responses consisted in the absence of the lemniscal and cortical components and preservation of waves generated at the brachial plexus and spine. Electroretinography was normal and visual evoked potential showed preservation of cortical components. 48 hours after admission (36 hours after the initial finding of brainstem areflexia) an apnoea test showed no breathing. Brainstem reflexes remained absent. Is this patient alive or dead?

Pallis (Pallis and Maggillivray, 1980; Pallis, 1983a; Pallis and Prior, 1983; Pallis, 1986, 1989, 1990a,b) proposed a standard that can also be separated according to the three main elements: definition, anatomical substratum and tests.

Definition

There is only one kind of human death: the irreversible loss of the capacity for consciousness, combined with the irreversible loss of the capacity to breathe (and hence to sustain a spontaneous heart beat).

For many centuries, respiration was considered the crucial function that defined the frontiers between life and death (Walker, 1981; Machado, 1994, 1995, pp. V–VI). In several ancient cultures death was considered: 'the departure of the soul from the body', and hence the words that stand for 'soul' are in many idioms the same as those standing for 'breath' (Pallis, 1986, 1990a,b).

Pallis postulated that the capacity for consciousness and respiration are two hallmarks of life for human beings, and that brainstem death predicts an inescapable asystole (Pallis and Maggillivray, 1980; Pallis, 1983a; Pallis and Prior, 1983; Pallis, 1989, 1990a).

Anatomical substratum
The permanent cessation of the functioning of the brainstem.

Pallis, (1990a) emphasized that the ascending reticular formation, discovered by Moruzzi and Magoun (1949) gives rise to a generalized activation of the cortex, producing the necessary arousal to endow the functioning of the 'brain as a whole'. He considered that the physiological and anatomical mechanism by which to abolish the capacity for consciousness is the irreversible damage of the paramedial tegmental areas of the mesencephalon and rostral pons.

Pallis also documented that the 'loss of breath' or apnoea relies on irreversible damage of the lower brainstem, where 'crucial mechanisms concerned with breathing are located' (Pallis, 1990a,b).

This author presented a detailed review to answer the question: How long may cardiac action persist after a diagnosis of brain death? He emphasized that in most cases asystole occurred within days, and that time variations in somatic survival after brain death presumably reflect three main factors: (1) the time on the ventilator before the diagnosis of brain death was made; (2) the quality of life support administered; and (3) the age of the individual (Pallis, 1990a).

Tests
According to Pallis (1986, 1990a,b) 'brainstem death is a clinical concept', and therefore 'a dead brainstem' can be diagnosed at the bedside. The procedure is to diagnose an unconscious patient, with irreversible apnoea and irreversible loss of brainstem reflexes, provided that 'all reversible causes of brainstem dysfunction have been excluded'.

Critique
Pallis (1990a) includes in his definition 'the capacity for consciousness', or arousal, as has been previously discussed. Nonetheless, in any definition that incorporates consciousness as a main hallmark, both components should be included, because normal conscious behaviour demands widespread interconnections among the ARAS, subcortical structures, and the neocortex, i.e. an interaction of both components (Plum, 1991; Machado, 1995, pp 57–66).

Moreover, some authors using deep brain stimulation have found non-specific cortical activation in PVS and comatose patients (Hassler *et al.*, 1969; Sturm *et al.*, 1979; Katayama *et al.*, 1991; Cohadon and Richer, 1993). Thus, in cases fulfilling the brainstem criteria of brain death with primary brainstem lesions and spared cerebral hemispheres, as in Case B, stimulation of the non-specific thalamic nuclei might produce some degree of arousal that could endow awareness. This would surely refute the diagnosis of brain death (Machado, 1995, pp. 57–66). In primary brainstem lesions a quasi-normal EEG could be recorded (Deliyannakis *et al.*, 1975; Ashwal and Schneider, 1979; Pallis, 1983b; Rodin *et al.*, 1985; Ferbert *et al.*, 1986).

Some recent reports have shown that some braindead patients do not develop an inevitable asystole within hours or days (Fabro, 1982; Kim *et al.*, 1982; Parisi *et al.*, 1982; Yoshiota *et al.*, 1986; Kinoshita *et al.*, 1990; Antonini *et al.*, 1992). Shewmon (1998b) has recently presented a detailed review of prolonged survivals in about 156 braindead patients. This author compiled cases with survival of more than 'a few days, i.e. one week or more', from sources including personal experience, the medical literature and the news media. He described a striking case of a patient with perhaps the longest recorded somatic survival, who was diagnosed (well documented) as 'braindead' 14½ years ago.

Shewmon (1998b) argued that the patient's age at onset of brain death plays a crucial role in somatic survival: 'the younger the age, the greater the capacity for survival'. This author also documented other factors implicated in survival: (1) 'associated systemic injuries directly due to whatever caused the brain insult'; and (2) 'systemic pathology secondarily induced by the process of brain herniation'. Withdrawal of life support is a 'confounding factor', because it can lead to an underestimate of the survival potential in braindead cases. The quality of nursing care, an adequate homeostatic control, prevention and early treatment of infections, etc., are other factors related to prolonged somatic survival. Consequently, an 'inevitable asystole' cannot be a justification for accepting a brain-oriented formulation of death.

THE HIGHER BRAIN STANDARD

Case C

HC was a 58-year-old female. She suffered a cardiorespiratory arrest due to a myocardial infarction. Reanimation manoeuvres took about 10 minutes. After complete recovery of normal cardiac activity, she remained deeply comatose and dependent on ventilatory assistance. In the acute phase, Babinski signs were present bilaterally and there was a transitory absence of pupillary, corneal and spinal reflexes. Repeat CT scans showed acute hydrocephalus, and an EEG taken during this phase did not reveal any electrical activity. The EEG remained isoelectric for the rest of survival. Brainstem auditory evoked components were preserved (I to V), although cortical short latency somatosensory and visual evoked potentials were absent. Three weeks after admission, she began to open her eyes and recovered sleep cycles; circulatory parameters were stable. In the fourth week, she did not need ventilatory assistance, breathing spontaneously, and she maintained an adequate control of body temperature. Liquefied food was placed directly into the stomach through a gastrostomy. Because she was incapable of moving on her own, she needed a special nursing care to prevent the development of bedsores. During her clinical evolution and for her next 12 years she was unable to understand anything at all; she could not communicate, and did not show any cognitive function. Is this patient alive or dead?

Definition
The loss of that which is significant to the nature of humans.

'Higher brain' advocates proposed defining death as 'the loss of that which is significant to the nature of man', (Mollaret and Goulon, 1959) and suggested that the irreversible loss of perception, sentience and cognition was necessary and sufficient for diagnosing death (Veatch, 1972, 1977, 1979; Green and Wikler, 1980; Puccetti, 1988; Wikler, 1988; Veatch, 1989; Cranford and Smith, 1990; Truog and Flacker, 1992; Wikler, 1995). Bartlett and Youngner (1988) asserted their belief 'that only the higher brain functions, consciousness and cognition, define the life and death of a human being'.

Robert M. Veatch, pioneer of this standard of death, argued for including in the definition 'capacity for consciousness or social interaction', and emphasized the presence in human beings of 'the functions considered to be ultimately significant to human life': rationality, consciousness, personal identity, and social interaction (Veatch, 1989). This author proposed that death should be properly defined 'as the irreversible loss of embodied capacity for social interaction'. Other authors have also proposed as the definition 'the loss of personhood' (Green and Wikler, 1980; Cranford and Smith, 1990).

Anatomical substraction
The permanent cessation of the functioning of the neocortex.

The defenders of this formulation sustained that the neocortex assumes a critical role to provide consciousness and cognition (Veatch, 1972; Bartlett and Youngner, 1988; Puccetti, 1988; Veatch, 1989). They functionally classified the brain into the lower brain (brainstem) that essentially controls vegetative functions, and the higher brain (the cerebral hemispheres, particularly the neocortex) that commands consciousness and cognition. Veatch (1989) also referred to the 'higher brain locus', or used other terms such as 'cerebral', 'cortical', or 'neocortical'. This author stated that 'we could be quite conservative and hold that the entire brain must be destroyed in order to be sure that the capacity for consciousness and social interaction is lost'.

Tests
No cognitive and affective functions.

Veatch clearly argued that elaborating a set of tests to measure the irreversible loss of the capacity for consciousness or social interaction is rather difficult.

Critique
As has been already discussed, arousal cannot simply be related to the function of the ARAS, and the content of consciousness related to the function of the

cerebral cortex, because substantial interconnections among the brainstem, subcortical structures and the neocortex are indispensable for both components of human consciousness (Plum and Posner, 1980; Plum, 1991; Machado, 1995, pp. 57–66. Hence, consciousness does not bear a simple one-to-one relationship with higher or lower brain structures, and the definition of consciousness does not correspond directly to the anatomical substratum (higher brain's anatomical locus). Unquestionably, the physical substratum for consciousness is based on anatomy and physiology throughout the brain. However the relationship is not simple (Machado, 1995, pp. 57–66).

Higher brain advocates have stressed that PVS cases are dead (Veatch, 1972, 1977, 1979; Green and Wikler, 1980; Bartlett and Youngner, 1988; Puccetti, 1988; Wikler, 1988; Veatch, 1989; Cranford and Smith, 1990; Truog and Flacker, 1992; Wikler, 1995). The main finding in PVS is the preservation of arousal with apparent loss of awareness (Machado, 1995, pp. 57–66). Kinney and Samuels (1994) emphasized that the PVS denotes a 'locked-out-syndrome', because the 'cerebral cortex is disconnected from the external world'. PVS occurs with one or more of three main neuropathological patterns: widespread and bilateral lesions of the cerebral cortex, diffuse damage of intra- and subcortical connections in the white matter of the cerebral hemispheres or necrosis of the thalamus.

Can we deny the existence of internal awareness in PVS, because these patients apparently seem to be disconnected from the external world? The subjective dimension of awareness is philosophically impossible to test, but physiologically it seems conceivable that subjective awareness might continue.

Karen Ann Quinlan's brain showed severe damage of the thalamus, with the cerebral hemispheres relatively spared (Kinney *et al.*, 1994). We can ask ourselves if, in a case like this, other activating pathways, projecting to the cerebral cortex without relaying through the thalamus, could stimulate the cerebral cortex to provide internal awareness, even if physicians are unable to detect its manifestations?

Unexpected and well-documented recoveries of cognitive functions have been described in patients diagnosed by neurologists experienced and skilled in the diagnosis of this condition (Rosenberg *et al.*, 1977; Steinbock, 1989; Childs *et al.*, 1993; Cohen-Almagor, 1997; Giacino, 1997). Childs *et al.* (1993) reported that 37% of 49 cases admitted to a special unit for rehabilitation were incorrectly diagnosed, according to the American Medical Association guidelines on PVS and the decision to withdraw support.

The use of deep brain stimulation showed that the cerebral hemispheres could mediate arousal, producing some wakefulness behaviour. This method has contributed to an undoubted recovery of awareness (recognition of their families and emotional expressions) in PVS patients (Hassler *et al.*, 1969; Sturm *et al.*, 1979; Katayama *et al.*, 1991; Cohadon and Richer, 1993).

Thus, in PVS cases it is impossible to deny a possible preservation of internal awareness. According to the neuropathological pattern, either subcortical structures could provide internal awareness, or some remaining activating pathways projecting to the cerebral cortex without relaying through the thalamus could stimulate the cerebral cortex (Machado, 1995, pp. 57–66). As consciousness is based on anatomy and physiology throughout the brain (Plum and Posner, 1980; Kinney and Samuels, 1994; Machado, 1995, pp. 57–66), it is impossible to classify a PVS case as dead. The brain is severely damaged, but consciousness may not be fully and irreversibly destroyed.

Moreover, it is necessary to consider the potential reversibility of awareness in PVS, as has been reported by some authors using deep brain stimulation (Hassler *et al.*, 1969; Sturm *et al.*, 1979; Katayama *et al.*, 1991; Cohadon and Richer, 1993). It is crucial to develop controlled multicentre studies to test and elaborate new protocols for sensory and pharmacological stimulation (Giacino, 1997). The possibility of brain function restoration in such patients, by current or as yet undeveloped techniques, is a challenge for the near future (Machado, 1994). In short, patient C is alive!

Thus, the main inconsistencies of the higher brain standard are:

(1) The definition of death does not correspond directly to the anatomical substratum, because proponents confuse the basis for consciousness with the neocortex.
(2) Proponents classify PVS cases as dead.

A NEW STANDARD OF HUMAN DEATH

Definition
Irreversible loss of consciousness which provides the key human attribute and the highest level of control in the hierarchy of integrating functions within the human organism.

Botkin and Post (1992) drew an interesting distinction between major and minor clusters of attributes related to life. For example, braindead patients retain several attributes associated with life, such as skin colour, warm skin, heartbeat, kidney function, etc. Even subjects who are dead according to the cardiorespiratory standard will preserve vestiges of life attributes for several days: hair and nails still grow (Pernick, 1988).

Cranford and Smith, 1990 stated 'our major premise is that consciousness is the most critical moral, legal, and constitutional standard, not for human life itself, but for human personhood'. Hence, higher brain defenders stressed that consciousness provides the most significant attribute of human existence (Veatch, 1979; Green and Wikler, 1980; Puccetti, 1988; Wikler, 1988; Cranford and Smith, 1990; Wikler, 1995). Therefore, the best candidate for the critical 'major attribute' of human life is consciousness: that is to say, without consciousness life loses most or all of its value for us. Consequently, I completely agree with higher brain advocates when considering that consciousness renders the most significant human attribute. Hence it is judicious to affirm that any vestige of consciousness is incompatible with death.

Korein (1977, 1997) defended the notion of integration, applying thermodynamics and information theory to living systems. He documented that all living organisms may be classified as open systems that exchange energy and matter with their environment. This author maintained that any organism contains a critical system which 'supersedes all other subsidiary systems' or subsystems. Korein suggested that the 'critical system' of the human organism is the brain. According to his view, therefore, if the brain is irreversibly destroyed, the critical system is abolished. Even if other subsystems are functioning spontaneously or supported by machines, the organism as an individual entity no longer exists.

The Swedish Committee on Defining Death (1985) also defended the notion of integration, defining death as: 'total and irreversible loss of all capacity for integrating and co-ordinating the functions of the body—physical and mental—into a functional unit'.

Shewmon (1985, 1992) had also been a defender of the central role of the brain 'in the coordination or performance of virtually all functions necessary for the unity of the post-embryonic human body, including internal homeostasis, adaptive interaction with the environment, and the intimate connection between mental and physiological states'. However, this author recently changed his position (1997, 1998a,b), when stating that the brain is not the 'central integrating organ of the body'. He stated that 'clinical evidence of brain death is more attributable to multisystem damage and spinal shock than to destruction of the brain per se', and proposed to return to a 'circulatory-respiratory' standard of death (Shewmon, 1997). However, this author accepted that the brain's plays a role in integrating the functions of the intact organism. He used as an example the field of psychoneuroimmunology, emphasizing that 'the brain role is one of modulating, fine tuning, and enhancing an already established and well functioning immune system'. If we accept Shewmon's view (1997, 1998a,b), then a specific emotional state could influence the immune system, either diminishing or enhancing the immune response. We can ask ourselves: Can we consider the brain's effect on other systems, of 'modulating' or 'fine-tuning' as 'the highest level of integration within the organism'?

Bernat (1991) affirmed that the brain generates signals 'for breathing through brainstem ventilatory centers, and aids in the control of circulation through medullary blood pressure control centers'. For example, if a young woman sees a flower with its connotations of beauty and love, or sees an assassin with a knife trying to attack her, the brain develops a complex control mechanism over the whole body. After visualizing and recognizing (backup memory) the visual target (flower or assassin), complex signals are generated through pathways that interconnect extensive brain areas (neocortex, diencephalon and other limbic structures, brainstem, reticular formation, etc.) producing faster heartbeats and deeper ventilatory movements (García *et al.*, 1995). Trained Yoga practitioners are capable of slowing heartbeats until they are almost imperceptible to auscultation (Telles *et al.*, 1995) The psychological influences in the menstrual cycle, and in reproduction, have been extensively discussed (Schou, 1998).

These examples demonstrate that consciousness controls and governs the functioning of the organism. This command over the organism can be conceived as 'modulating' or 'fine tuning', (Shewmon, 1997, 1998a,b) but it is, in fact, the highest level of control in the hierarchy of integrating functions within the human organism. Consciousness also stamps human individuality onto the integrated functioning of the body. Every subject responds in a different way to stimuli and daily life circumstances, according to his character, life experiences and personal interests.

This concept of consciousness as the ultimate integrative function is more consistent with the biologically based system concepts of Korein (1977, 1997) and Bernat *et al.* (Bernat, 1981; Bernat *et al.*, 1981, 1982; Guberman and Stuss, 1983; Bernat, 1984; Bernat *et al.*, 1984; Bernat, 1991, 1992a,b, 1998), than the more philosophically based notions of personhood favoured by Veatch (1972, 1977, 1979, 1989), Barlett and Youngner (1988), Wikler (Green and Wikler, 1980; Wikler, 1988; Kinoshita *et al.*, 1990) and others (Cranford and Smith, 1990; Truog and Flacker, 1992).

Anatomical substratum
Irreversible destruction of the anatomical and functional substratum of consciousness throughout the whole brain.

Substantial interconnections between the brainstem, subcortical structures and the neocortex are essential for subserving and integrating both components of human consciousness (Plum, 1991; Kinney and Samuels, 1994; Machado, 1994, 1995, pp. 57–66). Consequently, consciousness generation is based on anatomy and physiology throughout the brain.

Tests
Unresponsiveness, no arousal to any stimuli, and no cognitive and affective functions.

Implementing a reliable system to measure the irreversible loss of consciousness is quite difficult. The difficulty of obtaining physiological evidence of loss of consciousness is complicated by the philosophical difficulty of assessing the subjective dimension of consciousness (Bogen, 1997; Feinberg, 1997). Most sets of tests measuring the absence of brain functions demand evidence of unresponsiveness. This is mainly explored by applying painful stimuli (Beecher, 1968; Black, 1975; Walker, 1977; Guidelines, 1981; President's Commission, 1981; Guidelines, 1987; Machado *et al.*, 1991; Machado and García, 1995). Painful stimuli explore the arousal component of consciousness that activate cognitive and affective functions (Machado, 1995, pp. 57–66). Because the basis for consciousness is based on anatomy and physiology throughout the brain (Plum, 1991; Kinney and Samuels, 1994; Machado, 1995, pp. 57–66), sets of diagnostic criteria should include tests to evaluate both brainstem and cerebral hemispheres.

COMPARISON OF THE NEW STANDARD OF DEATH WITH OTHER STANDARDS (Table 17.1)

When this new standard of death is compared with whole brain, brainstem, and higher brain views, differences and similarities can be found.

Comparison with the whole brain standard
Similarities. Both views are based on anatomy and physiology throughout the brain. PVS cases are classified as alive.

Differences. In the new standard, only one function (consciousness) is considered as the hallmark of the definition rather than all functions of the brain.

Comparison with the brainstem standard
Similarities. In both views one of the components of consciousness is included as a hallmark (capacity for consciousness or arousal). PVS cases are classified as alive.

Differences. In the new standard, both components of consciousness are included as hallmarks. In the brainstem view, the brainstem alone is considered as the anatomical substratum.

Comparison with the higher brain standard
Similarities. In both views consciousness is considered as the hallmark for defining death.

Differences. In the higher brain standard, the neocortex alone is considered as the anatomical substratum, and PVS cases are classified as dead. The new standard identifies consciousness as the ultimate integrating function.

THOUGHT EXPERIMENT

To illustrate the new notion of human death, let us consider the following thought experiment.

Let us consider that we have all the technological wherewithal to substitute progressively all functions of a human being. When would this human become a robot? Which is the last function that could be replaced without abolishing the essential human attributes?

Let us suppose that Juan is a patient affected by a terminal metastatic cancer. Whenever a metastasis is found, the affected organ, function, or system is

Table 17.1 Comparison of different brain death standards

Standard	Definition	Anatomical substratum	Tests	Similarities with new view	Differences from new view
Whole brain	The permanent cessation of functioning of the organism as a whole	The permanent cessation of functioning of the entire brain	The permanent absence of breathing and heartbeat Brain cessation tests	Both views are based on anatomy and physiology throughout the brain PVS cases are classified as alive	In new view, only one function (consciousness) is considered as the hallmark of the definition rather than all functions of the brain
Brainstem	There is only one kind of human death: the irreversible loss of the capacity for consciousness, combined with the irreversible loss of the capacity to breathe (and hence to sustain a spontaneous heart beat)	The permanent cessation of functioning of brainstem	Irreversible apnoea and irreversible loss of brainstem reflexes, provided that 'all reversible causes of brainstem dysfunction have been excluded'	In both views one of the components of consciousness is included as a hallmark (capacity for consciousness or arousal) PVS cases are classified as alive	In new view both components of consciousness are included as hallmarks In the brainstem view, the brainstem alone is considered as the anatomical substratum (criterion)
Higher brain	The loss of that which is significant to the nature of humans	The permanent cessation of the functioning of the neocortex	No cognitive and affective functions	In both views consciousness is considered as the hallmark for defining death	In this view, the neocortex alone is considered as the anatomical substratum (criterion) PVS cases are classified as dead New definition identifies consciousness as the ultimate integrating function
New standard	Irreversible loss of the consciousness which provides the key human attribute and the highest level of control in the hierarchy of integrating functions within the human organism	Irreversible destruction of the anatomic and functional substratum of consciousness throughout the whole brain	Unresponsiveness, no arousal to any stimuli, and no cognitive and affective functions		

replaced by an artifice. In this way, the lungs, the heart, the stomach, the four limbs, are progressively substituted. The replacement will continue even into the brain. The visual pathways are completely substituted by specially designed electronic cameras; in the auditory system, electronic ears are wired into the brain. Eventually, the body is a complete electronic-mechanical artifice. All the brainstem, diencephalic, and other subcortical functions have been substituted. The only remaining functional structure is a unit formed by the activating reticular formation and the cerebral cortex, which is fully interconnected with the rest of the electronic brain and the artificial body. Is this 'electro-mechanic complex' a human?

If each replacement is perfect, the answer is: of course, it is a human being. The unit formed by the activating reticular formation and the cerebral cortex will still provide both components of consciousness, i.e. arousal and awareness. Nothing about Juan's personhood has changed: his thoughts, his memories, his affections, etc. Thus, the unit formed by the activating reticular formation and the cerebral cortex will maintain his essential human characteristics and will command and integrate the functioning of the rest of his 'electronic brain' and his 'artificial body'.

Let us now suppose that the unit formed by the activating reticular formation and the cerebral cortex could be surgically extracted from Juan's brain. Moreover, a special laboratory preparation provides the means to supply blood and oxygen to the unit. Is the preserved unit Juan? According to my theory the answer is: yes, it is Juan, because the unit conformed by the activating reticular formation and the cerebral cortex will still render both components of his conscious behaviour, i.e. arousal and awareness. This condition has to be considered as a combination of extreme locked-out and locked-in syndromes. Juan will be totally disconnected from the outer world, and he will not be able to express his thoughts and his feelings.

CONCLUSION

In conclusion, the best candidate for the critical 'major attribute' of human life is consciousness: that is to say, without consciousness life loses most or all of its value for us. Moreover, consciousness stamps human individuality on the integrated functioning of each of our bodies.

This essay proposes a standard of human death which identifies consciousness as the most important function of the body. It emphasizes that consciousness does not bear a simple one-to-one relationship with higher or lower brain structures, because the physical substratum for consciousness is based on anatomy and physiology throughout the brain.

Acknowledgements
I would like to thank Linda Emanuel and Adam Zeman for their careful reviews and precise suggestions during the elaboration of this paper.

REFERENCES

Antonini C, Alleva S, Campailla MT *et al.* (1992) Morte cerebrale e sopravvivenza fetale prolungata (Brain death and prolonged fetal survival). *Minerva Anestesiol* **58**:1247–1252.

Ashwal S and Schneider S (1979) Failure of electroencephalography to diagnose brain death in comatose patients. *Annals of Neurology* **6**:512–517.

Bartlett ET and Youngner SJ (1988) Human death and the destruction of the neocortex. In: *Death: Beyond the Whole-Brain Criteria* (ed. RM Zaner), pp. 199–215. New York: Kluwer.

Beecher HK (1968) A definition of irreversible coma: report of the Ad Hoc Committee of the Harvard Medical School to examine the definition of brain death. *Journal of the American Medical Association* **205**:85–88.

Bernat JL (1981) On the definition and criterion of death. *Annals of Internal Medicine* **94**:389–394.

Bernat JL (1984) The definition, criterion and statute of death. *Seminars in Neurology* **4**:45–51.

Bernat JL (1991) Ethical issues in neurology. In: *Clinical Neurology* (ed. RJ Joynt), pp. 1–105. Philadelphia: Lippincott.

Bernat JL (1992a) Brain death. Occurs only with destruction of the cerebral hemispheres and the brain stem. *Archives of Neurology* **49 (5)**:569–570.

Bernat JL (1992b) How much of the brain must die in brain death. *Journal of Clinical Ethics* **3**:21–28.

Bernat JL (1998) A defense of the whole-brain concept of death. *Hastings Center Report* **28**:14–23.

Bernat JL, Culver CM and Gert B (1981) Definition of death. *Annals of Internal Medicine* **95**:652.

Bernat JL, Culver CM and Gert B (1982) Defining death in theory and practice. *Hastings Center Report* **12 (1)**:5–8.

Bernat JL, Culver CM and Gert B (1984) Definition of death. *Annals of Internal Medicine* **100 (3)**:456.

Black PMcL (1975) Criteria of brain death. Review and comparison. *Postgraduate Medicine* **57**:69–74.

Bogen JE (1997) Some neurophysiological aspects of consciousness. *Seminars in Neurology* **17**:95–103.

Botkin JR and Post SG (1992) Confusion in the determination of death: Distinguishing philosophy from physiology. *Perspectives in Biology and Medicine* **36**:129–138.

Childs NL, Mercer WN and Childs HW (1993) Accuracy of diagnosis of persistent vegetative state. *Neurology* **43**:1465–1467.

Cohadon F and Richer E (1993) Stimulation cérébrale profonde chez des patients en état végétatif post-traumatique. 25 observations. *Neurochirurgie* **39**:281–292.

Cohen-Almagor R (1997) Some observations on post-coma unawareness patients and on other forms of unconscious patients: policy proposals. *Medicine and Law* **16**:451–47.

Conference of Royal Colleges and Faculties of the United Kingdom (1976) Diagnosis of brain death. *Lancet* **2**:1069–1070.

Conference of Royal Colleges and their Faculties of the United Kingdom (1979) Memorandum on the diagnosis of brain death. *British Medical Journal* **1**:322.

Cranford RE and Smith DR (1990) Consciousness: the most critical moral (constitutional) standard for human personhood. *American Journal of Law and Medicine* **332**:669–674.

Deliyannakis E, Ioannou F and Davaroukas A (1975) Brain-stem death with persistence of bioelectric activity of the cerebral hemispheres. *Clinical Electroencephalography* **6**:75–79.

Fabro F (1982) Brain death with prolonged somatic survival (Letter). *New England Journal of Medicine* **306**:1361.

Feinberg TE (1997) The irreducible perspectives of consciousness. *Seminars in Neurology* **17**:85–93.

Ferbert A, Buchner H, Ringelstein EB and Hacke W (1986) Isolated brain-stem death. Case report with demonstration of preserved visual evoked potentials. *Electroencephalography and Clinical Neurophysiology* **65**:157–160.

Fiser DH, Jimenez JF, Wrape V *et al.* (1987) Diabetes insipidus in children with brain death. *Critical Care Medicine* **15**:551–553.

García OD, Machado C, Román JM *et al.* (1995) Heart rate variability in coma and brain death. In: *Brain Death (Proceedings of the Second International Symposium on Brain Death)* (ed. C Machado), pp. 191–200. Amsterdam: Elsevier Science.

Giacino JT (1997) Disorders of consciousness: Differential diagnosis and neuropathological features. *Seminars in Neurology* **2**:105–111.

Green MB and Wikler D (1980) Brain death and personal identity. *Philosophy and Public Affairs* **2**:105–133.

Guberman A and Stuss D (1983) The syndrome of bilateral paramedian thalamic infarction. *Neurology* **33**:540–546.

Guidelines for the Determination of Brain Death (1981) Report of the Medical Consultants on the Diagnosis of Death to the President's Commission for the Study of Ethical Problems in Medicine and Biomedical and Behavioral Research. *Journal of the American Medical Association* **246**:2184–2186.

Guidelines for the determination of Brain Death in Children (1987) Report of the Task Force. *Neurology* **37**:1077–1078.

Hagl C, Szabo G, Sebening C, Tochtermann U, Vahl CF, Sonnenberg K and Hagl S (1997) Is the brain death related endocrine dysfunction and indication for hormonal substitution therapy in the early period? *European Journal of Medical Research* **2**:437–440.

Halery A and Brody B (1993) Brain death: reconciling definitions, criteria and tests. *Annals of Internal Medicine* **119**:519–525.

Hassler R, Dalle Ore G, Bricolo OA *et al.* (1969) Behavioral and EEG arousal induced by stimulation of unspecific projection systems in a patient with post-traumatic apallic syndrome. *Electroencephalography and Clinical Neurophysiology* **27**:306–310.

Howlett TA, Keogh AM, Perry L *et al.* (1989) Anterior and posterior pituitary function in brain-stem-dead donors. A possible role for hormonal replacement therapy. *Transplantation* **47**:828–834.

Jennett B (1981) Brain death (Editorial). *British Journal of Anaesthesiology* **53**:1111–1119.

Jennett B and Hessett C (1981) Brain death in Britain as reflected in renal donors. *British Medical Journal* **283**:359–362.

Katayama Y, Tsubokawa T, Yamamoto T *et al.* (1991) Characterization of brain activity with deep brain stimulation in patients in a persistent vegetative state: pain-related late positive component of cerebral evoked potential. *Pace* **14**:116–121.

Kim RC, Parisi JE, Collins GH and Hilfinger MF (1982) Brain death with prolonged somatic survival (Response to letter). *New England Journal of Medicine* **306**:1362–1363.

Kinney HC and Samuels MA (1994) Neuropathology of the persistent vegetative state: A Review. *Journal of Neuropathology and Experimental Neurology* **53**:548–558.

Kinney HC, Korein J, Panigraphy A, Dikkes P and Goode R (1994) Neuropathologic findings in the brain of Karen Ann Quinlan: The role of the thalamus in the persistent vegetative state. *New England Journal of Medicine* **330**:1469–1475.

Kinoshita Y, Yahata K, Yoshiota T *et al.* (1990) Long-term renal preservation after brain death maintained with vasopressin and epinephrine. *Transplant International* **3**:15–18.

Korein J (1977) The problem of brain death: Development and history. In: *Brain Death: Interrelated Medical and Social Issues* (ed. J Korein). New York: Annals of the New York Academy of Sciences **315**:19–38.

Korein J (1997) Ontogenesis of the brain in the human organism: definitions of life and death of the human being and person. In: *Advances in Bioethics*, Vol. 2 (ed. RB Edwards), pp. 1–74. New York: JAI Press.

Lugo N, Silver P, Nimkoff L, Caronia C and Sagy M (1997) Diagnosis and management algorithm of acute onset of central diabetes insipidus in critically ill children. *Journal of Pediatric Endocrinology and Metabolism* **10**:633–639.

Machado C (1994) Death on neurological grounds. *Journal of Neurosurgical Sciences* **38**:209–222.

Machado C, ed. (1995) *Brain Death (Proceedings of the Second International Symposium on Brain Death)*, pp. V–VI. Amsterdam: Elsevier Science.

Machado C and García A (1995) Guidelines for the determination of brain death. In: *Brain Death (Proceedings of the Second International Symposium on Brain Death* (ed. C Machado), pp. 75–80. Amsterdam: Elsevier Science.

Machado C, García-Tigera J, García OD, García-Pumariega J and Román JM (1991) Muerte Encefálica. Criterios diagnósticos. *Revista Cubana de Medicina* **30**:181–206.

Machado C, García OD, Román JM and Parets J (1995) Four years after the 'First International Symposium on Brain Death' in Havana: Could a definitive conceptual reapproach be expected? In: *Brain Death (Proceedings of the Second International Symposium on Brain Death)* (ed. C Machado), pp. 1–9. Amsterdam: Elsevier Science.

Molinari GF (1980) The NINCDS collaborative study of brain death: a historical perspective. In: *US Department of Health and Human Services, NINCDS Monograph No. 24*, NIH Publication No. 81–2226, pp. 1–32.

Mollaret P and Goulon M (1959) Le coma dépassé. *Revue Neurologique* **101**:3–15.

Moruzzi G and Magoun HW (1949) Brain stem reticular formation and activation of the EEG. *Electroencephalography and Clinical Neurophysiology* **1**:455–473.

Multi-Society Task Force on PVS (1994) Medical aspects of the persistent vegetative state. *New England Journal of Medicine* **330**:1499–1508.

Outwater KM and Rockoff MA (1984) Diabetes insipidus accompanying brain death in children. *Neurology* **34**:1243–1246.

Pallis C (1983a) Whole-brain reconsidered–physiological facts and philosophy. *Journal of Medical Ethics* **9**:32–37.

Pallis C (1983b) ABC of brain stem death. The arguments about the EEG. *British Medical Journal* **286**:284–287.

Pallis C (1986) Death. *Encyclopaedia Britannica*, Vol. 16, pp. 1030–1042.

Pallis C (1989) Death–beyond the whole-brain criteria. *Journal of Neurology, Neurosurgery and Psychiatry* **52**:1023–1024.

Pallis C (1990a) Brainstem death. In: *Handbook of Clinical Neurology: Head Injury* (ed. R Braakman), pp. 441–496. Amsterdam: Elsevier Science.

Pallis C (1990b) Brainstem death: the evolution of the concept. *Seminars in Thoracic and Cardiovascular Surgery* **2**:135–152.

Pallis C and Maggillivray B (1980) Brain death and the EEG. *Lancet* **2**:1085–1086.

Pallis C and Prior PF (1983) Guidelines for the determination of death. *Neurology* **33**:251–252.

Parisi JE, Kim RC, Collins GH and Hilfinger MF (1982) Brain death with prolonged somatic survival. *New England Journal of Medicine* **306**:14–16.

Pernick MS (1988) Back from the grave: Recurring controversies over defining and diagnosing death in history. In: *Death: Beyond the Whole-Brain Criteria* (ed. RM Zaner), pp. 17–74. New York: Kluwer.

Plum P (1991) Coma and related global disturbances of the human conscious state. In: *Cerebral Cortex*, Vol. 9 (ed. A Peters), pp. 359–425. New York: Plenum.

Plum F and Posner JB (1980) *The Diagnosis of Stupor and Coma*. Philadelphia: FA Davis.

President's Commission for the Study of Ethical Problems in Medicine and Behavioral Research (1981) *Defining Death. Medical Legal and Ethical Issues in the Determination of Death*. Washington, DC: US Government Printing Office.

Puccetti R (1988) Does anyone survive neocortical death? In: *Death: Beyond Whole-Brain Criteria* (ed. RM Zaner), pp. 75–90. Boston: Kluwer.

Rodin E, Tahir S, Austin D and Andaya L (1985) Brainstem death. *Clinical Electroencephalography* **16**:63–71.

Rosenberg GA, Johnson SF and Brenner RP (1977) Recovery of cognition after prolonged vegetative state. *Annals of Neurology* **2**:167–168.

Schou M (1998) Treating recurrent affective disorders during and after pregnancy. What can be taken safely? *Drug Safety* **18**:143–152.

Shewmon DA (1985) The metaphysics of brain death, persistent vegetative state, and dementia. *The Thomist* **49**:24–80.

Shewmon DA (1992) 'Brain death': A valid theme with invalid variations, blurred by semantic ambiguity. In: *Working Group on The Determination of Brain Death and its Relationship to Human Death* (eds H Angstwurm, I Carrasco de Paula), pp. 23–51. Vatican City: Pontificia Academia Scientiarum.

Shewmon A (1997) Recovery from 'brain death': a neurologist's apologia. *Linacre Quarterly*:30–96.

Shewmon DA (1998a) 'Brain-stem death', 'brain death' and death. A critical reevaluation of the purported equivalence. *Issues in Law and Medicine* **14(2)**:125–145.

Shewmon DA (1998b) Chronic 'brain death'. Meta-analysis and conceptual consequences. *Neurology* **51**:1538–1545.

Steinbock B (1989) Recovery from persistent vegetative state? The case of Carrie Coons. *Hastings Center Report* **19**:14–15.

Steriade M (1996) Arousal: revisiting the reticular activating system. *Science* **272**:225–226.

Sturm V, Kühner A, Schmitt HP, Assmus H and Stock G (1979) Chronic electrical stimulation of the thalamic unspecific activating system in a patient with coma due to midbrain and upper brain stem infarction. *Acta Neurochirurgica* **47**:235–244.

Swedish Committee on Defining Death (1985) *The Concept of Death. Summary.* Stockholm: Swedish Ministry of Health and Social Affairs.

Telles S, Nagarathna R and Nagendra HR (1995) Autonomic changes during 'OM' meditation. *Indian Journal of Physiology and Pharmacology* **39**:418–420.

Truog RD (1997) Is it time to abandon brain death? *Hastings Center Report* **27**:29–37.

Truog RD and Flacker JC (1992) Rethinking brain death. *Critical Care Medicine* **20**:1705–1713.

Veatch RM (1972) Brain death: welcome definition … or dangerous judgment? *Hastings Center Report* **11**:10–13.

Veatch RM (1977) The definition of death: ethical, philosophical, and policy confusion. In: *Brain Death: Interrelated Medical and Social Issues* (ed. J Korein). New York: Annals of the New York Academy of Sciences **315**:307–317.

Veatch RM (1979) Defining death: the role of brain function. *Journal of the American Medical Association* **242**:2001–2002.

Veatch RM, ed. (1989) Death, Dying, and the Biological Revolution. Our Last Responsibility. New Haven: Yale University Press.

Walker AE, ed. (1981) *Cerebral Death.* Baltimore: Urban & Schwarzenberg.

Walker AE (1977) An appraisal of the criteria of cerebral death. A summary statement. A collaborative study. *Journal of the American Medical Association* **237**:982–986.

Wertheimer P, Jouvet M and Descotes J (1959) A propos du diagnostic de la mort du système nerveux dans le comas avec arrête respiration traites par respiration artificielle. *Presse Medicale* **67**:87–88.

Wikler D (1988) Not dead, not dying? Ethical categories and the persistent vegetative state. *Hastings Center Report* **18**:41–47.

Wikler D (1995) Who defines death? Medical, legal and philosophical perspectives. In: *Brain Death (Proceedings of the Second International Symposium on Brain Death)* (ed. C Machado), pp. 13–22. Amsterdam: Elsevier Science.

Yoshiota T, Sugimoto H, Uenishi M *et al.* (1986) Prolonged hemodynamic maintenance by the combined administration of vasopressin and epinephrine in brain death: a clinical study. *Neurosurgery* **15**:565–567.

Index

213